# PSYCHIATRY SPECIALTY BOARD REVIEW FOR THE DSM-IV

# BRUNNER/MAZEL CONTINUING EDUCATION IN PSYCHIATRY AND PSYCHOLOGY SERIES

**Series Editor:** Gene Usdin, M.D.

This series provides comprehensive, state-of-the-art study guides to help those who are preparing for advanced examinations in psychiatry and psychology. Written by experts representing various areas of specialization, the guides are designed to be accurate, current, and accessible.

5. PSYCHIATRY SPECIALTY BOARD REVIEW FOR THE DSM-IV
John C. Duffy, M.D. and J. Bryce McLaulin, M.D.

4. PREPARATION FOR LICENSING AND BOARD CERTIFICATION EXAMINATIONS IN PSYCHOLOGY: The Professional, Legal, and Ethical Components, *Second Edition*
Robert G. Meyer, Ph.D.

3. CHILD AND ADOLESCENT PSYCHIATRY FOR THE SPECIALTY BOARD REVIEW
Robert L. Hendren, D.O.

2. NEUROLOGY FOR THE PSYCHIATRY SPECIALTY BOARD REVIEW
Leon A. Weisberg, M.D.

1. PSYCHIATRY SPECIALTY BOARD REVIEW
William M. Easson, M.D., and Nicholas L. Rock, M.D.

Brunner/Mazel Continuing Education in Psychiatry and Psychology Series, No. 5

# PSYCHIATRY SPECIALTY BOARD REVIEW FOR THE DSM-IV

**John C. Duffy, M.D.**
*Professor of Psychiatry*
*Division of Infant, Child, and Adolescent Psychiatry*
*Louisiana State University Medical Center*
*New Orleans, Louisiana*

**J. Bryce McLaulin, M.D.**
*Assistant Professor of Psychiatry*
*Louisiana State University Medical Center*
*New Orleans, Louisiana*

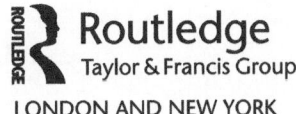 Routledge
Taylor & Francis Group

LONDON AND NEW YORK

First published 1996 by Brunner/Mazel, Inc.

Published 2020 by Routledge
2 Park Square, Milton Park, Abingdon, Oxon, OX14 4RN
52 Vanderbilt Avenue, New York, NY 10017

*Routledge is an imprint of the Taylor & Francis Group, an informa business*

Notice:
Product or corporate names may be trademarks or registered trademarks, and are used only for identification and explanation without intent to infringe.

**Note:** With dramatic advances continually being made in the clinical sciences, it is a challenge for physicians to keep abreast of both modifications in treatment that such advances require and of new drugs being introduced each year. The author and publisher of this volume have taken care to make certain that the doses of drugs and schedules of treatment are correct and compatible with the standards generally accepted at the time of publication. However, it is essential for the reader to become fully cognizant of the information on the instruction inserts provided with each drug or therapeutic agent prior to administration or prescription.

**Library of Congress Cataloging-in-Publication Data**

Duffy, John C. (John Charles)
    Psychiatry specialty board review for the DSM-IV/ John C. Duffy,
J. Bryce McLaulin.
      p.  cm. — (Brunner/Mazel continuing education in psychiatry
and psychology series ; no. 5)
    Includes bibliographical references.
    ISBN 0-87630-788-8 (pbk. : alk. paper)
    1. Psychiatry—Examinations, questions, etc.   I. McLaulin, J. Bryce.
II. Title.  III. Series.
    [DNLM: 1. Psychiatry—examination questions  2. Mental Disorders—
classification—examination questions.  3.  Certification—
examination questions.  WM 18.2 D858p 1996]
    RC457.D84  1996
    616.89'0076—dc 20
    DNLM/DLC
    for Library of Congress

95-26594
CIP

ISBN 13: 978-0-87630-788-5 (pbk)
ISBN 13: 978-1-138-46195-6 (hbk)

# CONTENTS

# SERIES EDITOR'S NOTE

As the fifth book in Brunner/Mazel's highly successful Continuing Education Series in Psychiatry and Psychology, this up-to-date study guide encompasses the important modifications in thinking introduced by the DSM-IV and recent advances in the field of biologic psychiatry. The book's format—multiple-choice, board-type questions and mock board examination questions with referenced answers—ensures easy access to information and accurate self-measurement in specific areas of study.

Drs. Duffy and McLaulin have done a superb job. This book will be an important aid to those preparing for their boards in psychiatry, as well as to those wanting a clear review and realistic evaluation of their current knowledge.

—GENE USDIN, M.D.
*Senior Psychiatrist, Ochsner Clinic*
*Clinical Professor of Psychiatry*
*Louisiana State University School of Medicine*
*New Orleans, Louisiana*

# PREFACE

At one time, board certification was an option for the psychiatrist. That time has passed. Certification is essential for the practice of psychiatry, and we likely soon will see a mandate for periodic recertification to maintain proof of competence and adequate knowledge of current diagnostics and treatments. This book can serve as an important tool in the preparation for the written examinations.

Psychiatry is undergoing momentous change: two powerful influences are the DSM-IV and recent developments in biologic psychology especially in psychopharmacology. Careful attention has been given to these areas, with all of the questions designed to reflect the latest information contained in the major reference books in the field. The questions, presented in examination format, and the instructive, detailed answers will help students to determine their level of knowledge and to supplement those areas in which there are gaps. Together with other aggressive study strategies, this book will lay the foundation for successful board examination preparation.

As the field of psychiatric research moves ahead, so too must its advocates, facilitators, pundits, recorders, and students. With this in mind, this book is also available on 3.5-inch disk, perhaps making it more convenient for those who are so inclined to use this versatile study guide.

JOHN C. DUFFY, M.D.
J. BRYCE McLAULIN, M.D.

# REFERENCES

Throughout this book, each question and chapter is referenced to one of three psychiatry text books. Rather than list each textbook and its authors with each reference, we have cited them as *DSM-IV, SP*, and *MCCAP* at the end of each answer.

DSM-IV: American Psychiatric Association. (1994). *Diagnostic and Statistical Manual of Mental Disorders* (4th ed.). Washington, D.C.: American Psychiatric Association.

SP: Kaplan, H. I., & Sadock, B. J. (1994). *Synopsis of Psychiatry* (7th ed.). Baltimore: Williams & Wilkins.

MCCAP: Robson, K. S. (1994). *Manual of Clinical Child & Adolescent Psychiatry* (rev. ed.). Washington, D.C.: American Psychiatric Association.

# 1

# CHILD AND ADOLESCENT PSYCHIATRY

# QUESTIONS

**DIRECTIONS: For questions 1 through 78, select the single best answer.**

1. Adoptive children:
   a. Are not remarkable in terms of incidence of emotional problems
   b. Tend to have lower IQ's than do nonadoptive children
   c. Have a high incidence of Attention-Deficit Hyperactivity Disorder
   d. In general have healthy life adjustments
   e. None of the above

2. According to recent theories, the way in which stimulant drugs may operate in Attention-Deficit Hyperactivity Disorder is:
   a. Paradoxical
   b. Sedative
   c. Nonspecific stimulation of the synaptic cleft
   d. Enhanced parasympathetic mechanism
   e. Central adrenergic mechanisms

3. Which is *not* a profile for an adolescent at risk for committing an agressive act?
   a. Is an older male adolescent
   b. Is of low socioeconomic status
   c. Has history of neurological impairment or learning disability
   d. Has history of drug or alcohol abuse
   e. Is oldest sibling in the family

4. Hospitalization in Anorexia Nervosa is:
   a. Psychiatric emergency
   b. Not recommended
   c. Requires long-term treatment
   d. None of the above

5. Anorexia Nervosa, Restricting Type, is characterized by:
   a. Severe reduction in caloric intake
   b. Refusal to maintain body weight
   c. Loss of more than 25% of original body weight
   d. Disturbances of body image
   e. All of the above

6. Which of the following is characteristic of Bulemic Anorexia Nervosa?
   a. No restriction of caloric intake
   b. Episodes of binge eating during Anorexia Nervosa
   c. Self-induced vomiting or use of laxitives or diuretics
   d. Affects multiple organ systems
   e. All of the above

7. A major effect of prolonged phenothiazine intake on psychotic and other hospitalized children is:
   a. Weight changes
   b. Tardive dyskensia
   c. Impaired learning
   d. Ocular changes
   e. All of the above

8. The prevalence of Infantile Autistic Disorder is:
   a. Two in 10,000
   b. Three in 10,000
   c. Four in 10,000
   d. Five in 10,000
   e. None of the above

9. Michael Rutter suggested that Autistic Disorder:
   a. Is psychodynamically conditioned
   b. Is strongly genetically influenced
   c. Has a high treatment success rate
   d. None of the above

10. Michael Rutter has defined the primary handicap in Autistic Disorder as:
    a. Defective superego
    b. Basic cognitive defect
    c. Maturational regression
    d. "System person"
    e. Pathological parents

11. Children who present with psychotic symptoms due to a General Medical Condition have:
    a. Long-term prodromal symptoms
    b. History of a precipitating emotional stress
    c. Family history of mental illness
    d. Visual hallucinations
    e. None of the above

12. Characteristics of sexual abuse in children include:
    a. Child is used for sexual gratification of an adult
    b. Child can also be abused by another child
    c. Is often progressive
    d. Usually involves secrecy
    e. All of the above

13. Common factors found in incestuous families include:
    a. Rape
    b. Ritualistic abuse
    c. False allegations
    d. Complex relationships with the offender that encompass more than just the abuse
    e. All of the above

14. A major problem in the diagnosis of sexual abuse in children is:

    a. Low consciousness of its prevalence
    b. Absence of physical signs, for example, genital or anal tears, bruises, or irritation
    c. Symptoms are nonspecific
    d. No history of overt violence
    e. None of the above

15–19. Match Erik Erikson's developmental stage with the proper achievement.

    a. Oral
    b. Anal
    c. Oedipal
    d. Latency
    e. Adolescent

15. Identity

16. Initiative

17. Trust

18. Autonomy

19. Industry

20. Bender Gestalt test result(s) suggestive of brain damage include:

    a. Directional confusion
    b. Inability to reproduce the gestalts
    c. Poor organization
    d. Perseveration
    e. All of the above

21. Which of the following is a major source of referral to child psychiatry?

    a. Physicians
    b. Schools
    c. Social agencies
    d. Courts
    e. Parents

22. An uncommon metabolic disorder that can present dual psychiatric symptoms is:

    a. Graves' Disease
    b. PKU
    c. Hartnup disease
    d. Critin's disease

23–27. Match each of Erik Erikson's following developmental achievements with its corresponding defect.

    a. Trust
    b. Industry
    c. Initiative
    d. Identity
    e. Autonomy

23. Shame, doubt

24. Mistrust

25. Inferiority

26. Guilt

27. Role defusion

28–31. Match each of Erik Erikson's following developmental achievements with its corresponding defect.

    a. Generative
    b. Intimacy
    c. Integrity
    d. Identity

28. Stagnation

29. Disgust, despair

30. Role

31. Isolation

32. The Wide Range Achievement Test includes:

    a. Letter and word recognition
    b. Spelling and writing
    c. Number and computational skills
    d. All of the above

33–36. Match the diagnostic condition with the appropriate IQ.

    a. 20–35 IQ
    b. 68–83 IQ
    c. Under 20 IQ
    d. 52–67 IQ
    e. 36–51 IQ

33. Borderline mental retardation

34. Mild mental retardation

35. Moderate mental retardation

36. Severe mental retardation

37. Which of the following is *not* a symptom of the antisocial personality?

    a. Intimate relationships
    b. No real feelings
    c. Inaccessibility
    d. Lack of concern
    e. Deceit and evasion

38–43. Match the following behavior problems with their age of manifestation.

a. Infancy to 2 years of age
b. Ages 3 to 5 years
c. Age 5 years and older
d. Ages 2 to 4 years
e. Ages 3 to 9 years

38. Feeding difficulties

39. Aggressiveness

40. Tics

41. Nodding spasms

42. Breath-holdings

43. Temper tantrums

44. Which of the following is *not* a function of the ego?

a. Drives
b. Relation to reality
c. Thought processes
d. Defensive functions
e. Synthetic functions

45. When young children present with behavioral disorders, among the important laboratory studies to be ordered are:

a. Lead
b. Glucose
c. Drug screen
d. Thyroid function

46. In Kallman's study of childhood Schizophrenia, the concordance rate for identical twins was:

a. 66%
b. 77%
c. 88%
d. 99%
e. None of the above

47. There is a suggestion that Schizophrenia may be localized on chromosome:

a. 4
b. 5
c. 6
d. 7
e. 8

48. Freud (1914) referred to the psychodynamics of parental love as:

a. Repression of unsocialized aggressive drives
b. Necessary for adult sexual maturity
c. Unrelated to psychosocial development
d. Projection of infantile self-love
e. None of the above

49–52. Match the person with his or her contribution.

a. Heimy Hartmann
b. Karl Abraham

c. J. C. Flugel
d. A. Freud

49. Structural period of psychoanalysis

50. Pregenital phases of development

51. Ego psychology and adaptation

52. Interpersonal structure of the family (psychoanalytic)

53. Margaret Mead is best known for her:

a. Comparative, empirical studies on the cultural basis of childhood socialization
b. Study of sexual development
c. Study of adolescent behavior
d. Study of attitude formation
e. All of the above

54. Drug used in the treatment of the Attention-Deficit Hyperactivity Disorder is:

a. Stelazine
b. Methylphenidate
c. Haldol
d. Clonidine
e. None of the above

55. The child, described by Freud in *From The History Of Infantile Neurosis* (1918), who at age $1\frac{1}{2}$ observed parental coitus, by the age 4 had developed

a. Schizophrenia
b. Separation anxiety
c. Phobia
d. Night terrors

56. The incidence of Nocturnal Enuresis in a child after seven years of age is:

a. One out of four
b. One out of five
c. One out of six
d. One out of seven
e. None of the above

57. Drug used most often in the successful treatment of Gilles de la Tourette's Disorder is:

a. Butyrophenones
b. Piperacetazine
c. Chlorpromazine
d. Mesoridazine
e. None of the above

58–60. Match the following neuromuscular movements with their appropriate names.

a. General motor restlessness
b. Chorea
c. Athetosis

58. Wormlike, continuous

59. Random, varied, and voluntary

60. Generalized large muscle groups

61. Direct murders of children are committed mostly by:

    a. Psychotic parent or relative
    b. Normal parent
    c. Person unrelated to the child
    d. Neighbor or friend of the family

62. In Harry Harlow's studies, unmothered monkeys raised by surrogates exhibited:

    a. Apathy
    b. Withdrawal
    c. Difficulty in learning to mate
    d. Difficulty in caring for their young
    e. All of the above

63. The so-called tormented child is one who is exposed to:

    a. Slapping and spanking during routine care giving
    b. Burns with cigarettes
    c. Minor lacerations
    d. Severe pinching
    e. All of the above

64. Adelaide Johnson and S. Szurek developed an explanation of antisocial acting out in children based on:

    a. Psychosocial regression
    b. Poor ego control
    c. "Superego lacone"
    d. Inconsistent mothering
    e. Having a single parent

65. Major factor in parents' management of children during World War II that diminished anxiety was:

    a. Frank communication of danger
    b. Overt expression of fear
    c. Ignoring of danger
    d. Removal of child from the parents
    e. Placement of the child away from the danger zone

66. Rene Spitz identified damaging maternal behavior patterns as:

    a. Primary overt rejection
    b. Primary anxiety and overt permissiveness
    c. Oscillation between pampering and hostility

    d. Cyclical mood swings of the mother
    e. All of the above

67–70. Match the most likely diagnosis presenting as intellectual progressive deterioration with the appropriate age group.

    a. Infancy up to 5 years
    b. Childhood, 6 to 16 years

67. Diffuse sclerosis (Schilder's)

68. Degeneration (Tay-Sachs)

69. Subdural hematoma

70. Tuberous sclerosis

71. Anorexia Nervosa was named by:

    a. Levy
    b. Cabot
    c. Bender
    d. Gull
    e. Spitz

72. A major treatment modality for school refusal in a child is:

    a. Tutoring at home
    b. Removal from the home
    c. Immediate return to school
    d. Hospitalization

73–78. Match the activity on the electroencephologram with the most likely etiology.

    a. Hypsarrahythmia
    b. Diffuse, bilateral spike and wave
    c. Six-per-second and 14-per-second positive spike discharge

73. Petit mal epilepsy

74. Recurrent headaches, abdominal pain, autonomic dysfunction

75. Normal children

76. Minor motor epilepsy

77. Recurrent frequency varying from $2\frac{1}{2}$ to 4 per second

78. Random low-voltage spike waves with slow (large) waves

# ANSWERS AND EXPLANATIONS

1. Answer is **d**. The emotional development of adoptees within their families (especially adoptees with traumatic histories) is often troubled to some extent. But from a psychological point of view the majority of all adoptees do quite well in the long run. *(MCCAP 396)*

2. Answer is **c**. The general consensus is that stimulants prevent catecholamine reuptake at the synaptic cleft, as well as inhibit metabolism and breakdown. *(MCCAP 226)*

3. Answer is **e**. Research on teenagers who have committed serious crimes indicates a number of risk factors. Among the more serious are a strong drive to be violent and easy access to a weapon. *(MCCAP 262)*

4. Answer is **a**. Children with eating disorders often present as psychiatric emergencies. This is so because of their high morbidity and mortality. Therefore, it is essential that the psychiatrist and emergency room personnel be familiar with this condition and its high risk for a fatal outcome. *(MCCAP 278)*

5. Answer is **e**. There are two subcategories of eating disorders: Anorexia Nervosa, Restricting Type, and Bulimic Anorexia Nervosa. They present as different entities in terms of their symptom complex. *(MCCAP 278)*

6. Answer is **e**. The patient presenting with a symptom complex of Bulemic Anorexia Nervosa is characterized by a restriction of caloric intake alternating with episodes of binge eating and vomiting. *(MCCAP 278)*

7. Answer is **e**. All of the major phenothiazines function as dopamine, α-adrenergic blockers in the central nervous system and peripheral nervous system. Over time, the incidence of side effects increases dramatically and should be a major concern before initiating treatment over a longer-term period with children. *(MCCAP 221–222)*

8. Answer is **c**. Autistic Disorder is a relatively rare condition with a population prevalence of 4 in 10,000 or 0.04%. *(MCCAP 422)*

9. Answer is **b**. A number of studies by Rutter and Folstein on monozygotic twins found the genetic rate to be approximately 15%. Since the base rate is so low for Autistic Disorder in the general population, Rutter has strongly suggested that it is one of the most genetically influenced psychiatric conditions in children. *(MCCAP 422)*

10. Answer is **b**. The most important deficit for the child with Autistic Disorder concerns the inability to cope on a cognitive level, which results in extreme social disability. *(MCCAP 422)*

11. Answer is **d**. A child with a Psychotic Disorder due to a General Medical Condition is unique in that the onset is very recent, there is no history of an emotional stress, the family has no prior mental illness, and frequently the hallucinations are visual rather than the more characteristic auditory hallucinations of Schizophrenia. *(MCCAP 271)*

12. Answer is **e**. Sexual abuse covers the widest range of activities in which a child is used for sexual gratification by an adult, as well as another child. If the perpetrator is significantly older than the victim, that is, at least five years or more older, it is often progressive in that it may begin as cuddling, and then go on to genital touching. Secrecy is a major factor, often involving threats to the life of the child. *(MCCAP 286)*

13. Answer is **e**. Factors that seem to be very common in families in which incest occurs and so should alert the clinician as to the possibility of incest, are reported incidents of rape or ritualistic abuse, such as seen in some cults or in groups involved in satanic worship, and false allegations of sexual abuse of the child in divorce or custody disputes in which one party seeks to gain custody over the other party. *(MCCAP 287)*

14. Answer is **a**. Sexual abuse will be recognized by the clinician as part of the differential diagnosis only when his or her consciousness has been raised to the point that the clinician appreciates that there is a very real prevalence of the condition, resulting in multiple serious psychological sequela. *(MCCAP 291)*

15. Answer is **e**.

16. Answer is **c**.

17. Answer is **a**.

18. Answer is **b**.

19. Answer is **d**.

Erikson conceived of development as a series of specific tasks conforming to more or less identified periods of childhood and adolescence. If there was failure in any stage, then this for him represented "unfinished business." For example, an infant who fails to establish basic trust in the first year of life will be plagued by distrust in later relationships. *(MCCAP 4)*

**20.** Answer is **e**. The Bender Gestalt has been in use by clinicians since the 1930s. It is made up of nine classic geometric designs that the child has to copy on paper. The skill and ability to do this is then used as an indicator of maturational growth and level, and also of the possibility of organic dysfunction. *(MCCAP 80)*

**21.** Answer is **b**. There is no question that the school is a major source of referral to child psychiatry. The reason is that it is a social and learning situation in which the child, who might otherwise be protected at home or not thought to be handicapped by the physician, clearly evinces developmental and/or behavioral disorders that make their appearance in the classroom. *(MCCAP 38)*

**22.** Answer is **c**. Hartnup Disease is a rare metabolic disorder associated with high levels of amino acids in the urine, specifically threonine, tyrosine, and histidine. *(MCCAP 47)*

**23.** Answer is **e**.

**24.** Answer is **a**.

**25.** Answer is **b**.

**26.** Answer is **c**.

**27.** Answer is **d**.

When a developmental achievement is met with a defect, that failure creates future psychological problems for the individual. *(MCCAP 4)*

**28.** Answer is **a**.

**29.** Answer is **c**.

**30.** Answer is **d**.

**31.** Answer is **b**.

When a developmental achievement is associated with a defect, these are the types of problems that result. *(MCCAP 4)*

**32.** Answer is **d**. The Wide-Range Achievement Test was developed for Jastak and Wilkinson in 1984. It includes brief screening measures for letters and word recognition, spelling and writing, and number and computational skills. The age range for this examination is K to post-12th grade. *(MCCAP 78)*

**33.** Answer is **b**.

**34.** Answer is **d**.

**35.** Answer is **e**.

**36.** Answer is **a**.

Normative data from most tests have been statistically manipulated such that an IQ of 100 is average. Scores that differ from the mean by more than one standard deviation (in either direction) are considered to be significant and thereby indicative of relative strengths or weaknesses. *(MCCAP 78)*

**37.** Answer is **a**. By late adolescence many of the cardinal symptoms of the psychopathic personality are in evidence. One of the two hallmarks of this condition is the seeming inability to form intimate relationships. *(MCCAP 83)*

**38.** Answer is **a**.

**39.** Answer is **b**.

**40.** Answer is **c**.

**41.** Answer is **a**.

**42.** Answer is **d**.

**43.** Answer is **e**.

One of the most critical issues in understanding the behavioral disorders of children is whether the problem is age appropriate or inappropriate. There can be clusters of disorders of behavior that are normal at one stage in a child's life, but at another age have to be considered abnormal. *(MCCAP 178)*

**44.** Answer is **a**. Among the many important functions of the ego, drives are not part of its process. *(MCCAP 7)*

**45.** Answer is **a**. Lead exposure is a frequent finding in young children from poor socioeconomic environments. A level as high as 40 $\mu$g is seen as within the normal range. However, most clinicians are concerned with a blood level above 15. It is almost always associated with behavioral problems. *(MCCAP 46)*

**46.** Answer is **c**. Many studies have validated Kallman's original concordance rate for this disease. There is very little support for a single major-locus genetic type of inheritance. Linkage studies are preliminary and currently inconsistent. There is some thought that it is a heterogeneous condition. *(MCCAP 424)*

**47.** Answer is **b**. Localization on chromosome 5 was suggested by McGilivray in 1990; however, this has not been verified in follow-up studies. *(MCCAP 423)*

48. Answer is **d**. Freud's insight was important in that he equated the success of a parent's love for a child with the successful achievement of his or her own infantile self-love and the ability to project it on the child. *(MCCAP 4)*

49. Answer is **d**.

50. Answer is **b**.

51. Answer is **a**.

52. Answer is **c**.

These persons played significant early roles in formulating the psychoanalytic concept of the development of the child. *(MCCAP 4)*

53. Answer is **e**. Margaret Mead identified and carried forward the psychoanalytic concepts of the role of culture in childhood socialization. This was related to issues around sexual, adolescent, and attitude development. *(MCCAP 13)*

54. Answer is **b**. Methylphenidate (Ritalin) is the drug of choice in the treatment of Attention-Deficit Disorder. Of all of the stimulants and other medications, it has had the highest success rate. *(MCCAP 115)*

55. Answer is **c**. In this landmark report, Freud identified the origins of phobia as a displacement from exposure to an acute anxiety-provoking incident to another less-threatening experience. *(MCCAP 248)*

56. Answer is **a**. Enuresis, particularly in young males, is often a troublesome symptom. It may or may not be related to a neurotic condition. Physical symptoms, such as a small bladder or spasm of the bladder muscle, needs to be ruled out. *(MCCAP 231)*

57. Answer is **e**. The initial and most successful treatment regimen for Tourettes Disorder is haloperidol beginning with 0.25 mg for three to four days, then increasing the dosage by 0.25 mg every five to seven days. If this fails to control the symptoms a number of other drugs are tried. *(MCCAP 225)*

58. Answer is **c**.

59. Answer is **a**.

60. Answer is **b**.

It is important in treating young children with major psychotropic agents to be able to distinguish various movements and whether or not they might be related to the medication. *(MCCAP 439)*

61. Answer is **a**. In incidents of child murder, it is typical to find that a parent, very often the mother, is suffering from a major psychotic condition that is directly responsible for her motives for murdering the child. *(MCCAP 298)*

62. Answer is **e**. Dr. Harlow's studies with monkeys verified what was intuitively understood in clinical situations, that is, that the absence of a mothering figure results in serious adjustment problems. *(MCCAP 321)*

63. Answer is **e**. This is a syndrome that often is unrecognized in terms of child abuse, and yet, in many respects, results in the same serious psychopathology. It is important in taking a history to identify whether or not spanking or slapping is used in caregiving, and, of course, a physical examination will reveal evidence of burns, pinching, or lacerations. *(MCCAP 239)*

64. Answer is **c**. Johnson and Szurek proposed that, similar to Swiss cheese, there are "holes" in the child's superego that through parental support, encourage antisocial acting out. *(MCCAP 198)*

65. Answer is **a**. During World War II, when children in Europe were at risk, parents had the greatest success when they were comfortable with communicating to the children the realistic aspect of the danger of being in a war situation. *(MCCAP 234)*

66. Answer is **e**. Spitz was one of the early researchers who identified those aspects of the mother that create the greatest risk for serious psychopathology in the infant. *(MCCAP 341)*

67. Answer is **b**.

68. Answer is **a**.

69. Answer is **a**.

70. Answer is **a**.

Of all four of these conditions, subdural hematoma is reversible if correctly diagnosed early in the course of the conditions. The other conditions are genetic with major deterioration of intelligence and death. *(MCCAP 414–420)*

71. Answer is **d**. This condition was first described by Gull. His description of the symptoms is as accurate today as when he first reported them. *(MCCAP 36)*

72. Answer is **c**. The first and most important approach to this problem is to insist that the parent assure that the child will return to school immediately. When this fails, there are important psychopharmacological treatments that seem to improve the chances of the successful return of the child to school. *(MCCAP 231)*

73. Answer is **b**.

74. Answer is **c**.

75. Answer is **c**.

76. Answer is **a**.

77. Answer is **c**.

78. Answer is **a**.

The EEG can be a valuable tool in the initial diagnostic evaluation of a variety of conditions that may present as behavioral but may have neurological origins. *(MCCAP 321)*

# 2
# PSYCHOPATHOLOGY

# QUESTIONS

**DIRECTIONS: For questions 1 through 105, select the single best answer.**

1. All of the following statements about Delirium are true **EXCEPT:**
   a. Children may be especially susceptible to delirium.
   b. The elderly are most vulnerable to delirium.
   c. Ten percent of individuals over age 65 hospitalized for a medical condition have delirium.
   d. Disorientation to self is common in delirious patients.
   e. Frightening visual hallucinations may be a prominent symptom in delirious patients.

2. When differentiating Delirium from other conditions or disorders, all of the following statements are true **EXCEPT**:
   a. Laboratory studies are important in this differential diagnosis process.
   b. Preexisting dementia will increase the vulnerability of a patient to the development of Delirium.
   c. The psychotic symptoms of Delirium are indistinguishable from those of other psychotic disorders.
   d. The inability to focus and shift attention is important in the differential diagnosis process.
   e. Malingering and Factitious Disorder must be included in the differential diagnosis.

3. All of the following must be present for a diagnosis of Dementia **EXCEPT:**
   a. Memory impairment
   b. Disturbance in level of consciousness
   c. Aphasia, agnosia, or apraxia
   d. Disturbance in executive function
   e. Deficits representing a decline from previous level of functioning

4. Diagnostic criteria for Amnestic Disorder in DSM-IV include all of the following **EXCEPT:**
   a. Apraxia, aphasia, and disturbance of executive function are prominent in this disorder.
   b. Patients with Amnestic Disorder have an impaired ability to learn new information.
   c. The memory disturbance in affected individuals is severe.
   d. Disorientation to self is unusual in Amnestic Disorder.
   e. Patients with Amnestic Disorders frequently have no insight into their memory deficit and will deny even severe deficits.

5. Criteria used by DSM-IV for the differentiation of primary mental disorder from a Mental Disorder Due to a General Medical Condition include all of the following **EXCEPT:**
   a. Presence of a medical disorder.
   b. Physiological mechanism links the psychiatric symptomatology to the general medical condition.
   c. Disturbance not accounted for by another mental disorder.
   d. Presence of features atypical of a primary mental disorder.
   e. All of the above.

6. Which of the following statements is/are true of the DSM-IV diagnosis Personality Change Due to a General Medical Condition?
   a. Cognitive decline is a feature of diagnosis.
   b. Personality disturbance represents a deviation from the individual's previous personality pattern.
   c. Patient may exhibit affective lability, poor impulse control, and outbursts of aggression.
   d. Personality change is due to the direct physiological effects of a medical disorder.
   e. Discriminating factor between this diagnosis and a Mental Disorder Due to a General Medical Condition is that the deviation from a previously stable personality structure is most prominent.

7. Correct statements about DSM-IV diagnosis of Substance Abuse include all of the following **EXCEPT:**
   a. Diagnosis does not apply to caffeine or nicotine.
   b. Recurrent Substance Abuse resulting in a failure to fulfill major role obligations, being placed in physically hazardous situations, or incurring legal problems characterizes this diagnosis.
   c. Diagnosis does not include tolerance or withdrawal.
   d. Diagnosis of Substance Abuse and Substance Dependence are not mutually exclusive.
   e. Problems related to Substance Abuse must be recurrent over a 12-month period.

8. All of the following statements regarding Schizophrenia are true **EXCEPT:**
   a. Auditory hallucinations are the most common and characteristic hallucinations in patients with Schizophrenia.
   b. Patients with schizophrenia cannot differentiate auditory hallucinations from their own thoughts.
   c. Pejorative or threatening voices are common.
   d. One or more voices keeping a running commentary on the patient's behavior will fully satisfy the thought-disorders criterion for Schizophrenia.
   e. Hypnagogic and hypnopompic hallucinations are considered within the realm of normal experience and not part of a schizophrenic process.

9. All of the following statements according to DSM-IV

regarding the effects of Schizophrenia on speech and behavior are true **EXCEPT**:

a. Clinical inferences about thought processes are based primarily on the patient's speech pattern.
b. Goal-directed behavior may be especially problematic for patients with Schizophrenia.
c. Speech is significantly impaired so as to impede effective communication.
d. According to DSM-IV, aimless and seemingly purposeless behavior must be distinguished from grossly disorganized behavior.
e. Catatonic behaviors occur exclusively in patients with Schizophrenia.

10. According to DSM-IV, which of the following may be the best predictor of poor outcome for an individual with Schizophrenia?

a. Lack of insight
b. Difficulty in concentrating
c. Affective symptoms
d. Sleep disturbance
e. Somatic delusions

11. Risk factors for suicide in individuals with Schizophrenia include all of the following **EXCEPT**:

a. Male gender
b. Being over 30 years old
c. Depressive symptoms
d. Being unemployed
e. Recent hospital discharge

12. DSM-IV requires a longer time of active symptomatology for the diagnosis of Schizophrenia than did DSM-III-R. By what factor has it been increased?

a. Times two
b. Times three
c. Times four
d. Times five
e. Times six

13. According to DSM-IV, all of the following statements regarding Schizophrenia are true **EXCEPT**:

a. The age of onset of Schizophrenia is typically between the late teens and early 30s.
b. Women are more likely to have a later onset.
c. The lifetime prevalence is usually estimated to be between 0.5% and 1%.
d. First-degree biological relatives of individuals with Schizophrenia have a risk for Schizophrenia that is 25 times greater than in the general population.
e. Hospital-based studies suggest a higher rate of Schizophrenia for males, whereas community-based studies suggest an equal sex ratio.

14. DSM-IV lists differences between late-onset (>45 years) Schizophrenia and the more typical early-onset type. All

of the following statements about this difference are true **EXCEPT**:

a. A higher ratio of women have late-onset Schizophrenia.
b. Negative symptoms and disorganized thinking are more common in late-onset Schizophrenia.
c. A better occupational history is associated with late-onset Schizophrenia.
d. The clinical presentation of late-onset Schizophrenia is more likely to include paranoid delusions and hallucinations.
e. The course of late-onset Schizophrenia tends to be chronic.

15. Characteristics of the Paranoid Type of Schizophrenia listed in DSM-IV include all of the following **EXCEPT**:

a. Prominent delusions and/or hallucinations are the essential features of the Paranoid Type of Schizophrenia.
b. Delusions are typically organized around a coherent type and are often grandiose or persecutory.
c. The prognosis for the Paranoid Type of Schizophrenia may be better than for other types of Schizophrenia.
d. The distinguishing characteristics of the Paranoid Type of Schizophrenia tend to fluctuate over time.
e. Individuals with the Paranoid Type of Schizophrenia may be haughty, aloof, or very formal in their interactions.

16. All of the following represent DSM-IV criteria for the diagnosis of Schizophrenia of the Catatonic Type **EXCEPT**:

a. Cataplexy
b. Excessive motoric activity
c. Extreme negativism
d. Posturing
e. Echolalia or echopraxia

17. All of the following statements represent DSM-IV criteria for Delusional Disorder **EXCEPT**:

a. One or more nonbizarre delusions are present for one month.
b. Mood disturbances are often prominent in this disorder.
c. The diagnoses of Schizophrenia and Delusional Disorder are mutually exclusive.
d. Tactile and olfactory hallucinations may be prominent if they are related to the delusional theme.
e. If present, auditory and visual hallucinations are not prominent.

18. Types of Delusional Disorder include all of the following **EXCEPT**:

a. Hypochondriacal type
b. Erotomanic type
c. Jealous type
d. Mixed type
e. Grandiose type

19. Which of the following statements regarding Shared Psychotic Disorder is true?

    a. The shared delusional system develops in the affected individuals concurrently over a period of time.

    b. When the affected persons are separated, both will maintain the delusions developed by the pair.

    c. The shared delusions are almost always of a persecutory nature.

    d. Usually one of the pair begins this process as a healthy, although passive, individual.

    e. For this diagnosis, neither of the pair can be diagnosed as having Schizophrenia.

20. All of the following statements about Major Depressive Episode as defined by DSM-IV are true **EXCEPT**:

    a. Sleep disturbance occurs almost every day.

    b. Fatigue or loss of energy occurs almost every day.

    c. Decreased interest in pleasurable activities occurs nearly every day.

    d. Ability to pay attention or concentrate is decreased.

    e. Duration of depressive symptoms must be at least four weeks to meet criteria.

21. A Manic Episode:

    a. Must last at least one week (or less if hospitalization is required) to meet criteria.

    b. Is rarely preceded or followed by a depressive episode.

    c. Usually does not involve symptoms of a psychotic nature.

    d. Usually results in the patient's spontaneously seeking psychiatric care.

    e. By definition, never has concurrent depressive symptoms.

22. The Hypomanic Episode (DSM-IV):

    a. Is a distinct period during which there is an abnormally and persistently elevated, expansive, or irritable mood that lasts at least one week.

    b. Does not require that mood or behavioral changes be observed by others for diagnosis.

    c. Always results in social or occupational impairment.

    d. Cannot include delusions or hallucinations as a part of this clinical picture.

    e. Is not clearly distinct from the individual's usual non-depressed function and mood.

23. All of the following statements regarding Major Depressive Disorder are true **EXCEPT**:

    a. The lifetime risk for Major Depressive Disorder in men is 5% to 12 %.

    b. Prevalence rates for this disorder are highly correlated with ethnicity, education, income, or marital status.

    c. Some 15% of individuals with severe Major Depressive Disorder kill themselves.

    d. The disorder is twice as common in adolescent and adult females as in adolescent and adult males.

    e. Up to 25% of individuals with chronic medical conditions develop Major Depressive Disorder.

24. All of the following statements about the course of illness of Major Depressive Disorder are true **EXCEPT**:

    a. The severity of an initial episode of Major Depressive Disorder does not predict the persistence of depressive symptoms.

    b. Episodes of Major Depressive Disorder often follow a severe psychosocial stressor.

    c. According to follow-up national studies, one year after the diagnosis of Major Depressive Disorder, 40% of individuals still meet the criteria for Major Depressive Episode.

    d. Partial remission following an episode increases the likelihood of developing additional episodes.

    e. This disorder is $1\frac{1}{2}$ to three times more common in first degree biological relatives than in the general population.

25. All of the following statements regarding Dysthymic Disorder are true **EXCEPT**:

    a. The essential feature is a chronically depressed mood for most of the day for two years.

    b. For DSM-IV diagnosis, in addition to two years of depressed mood, two additional depressive symptoms such as appetite disturbance, low self-esteem, or sleep disturbances, must be present.

    c. The patient experiences the depressive mood as ego-alien and uncharacteristic of his or her normal feeling state.

    d. Dysthymic Disorder has a lifetime prevalence of 6%.

    e. Subjective emotional symptoms dominate the symptom pattern in individuals with Dysthymic Disorder.

26. All of the following statements regarding Bipolar I Disorder are true **EXCEPT**:

    a. More than 90% of individuals who have a single Manic Episode go on to have future episodes.

    b. Some 60% to 70% of Manic Episodes occur immediately before or after a Major Depressive Episode.

    c. The first episode of this disorder in males is more likely to be a Major Depressive Episode.

    d. Women with this disorder have an increased risk of developing subsequent episodes in the postpartum period.

    e. Bipolar I Disorder with Rapid Cycling means four or more episodes per year.

27. All of the following statements about Cyclothymic Disorder are true **EXCEPT**:

    a. This diagnosis can only be made after two years of cyclothymic symptoms that are free of Major Depressive Manic, or Mixed Episodes.

    b. If a patient develops a Manic Episode after two years of cyclothymic symptoms, the diagnosis is Cyclothymic Disorder and Bipolar I Disorder.

    c. If a patient develops a Major Depressive Episode after two years of cyclothymic symptoms, the diagnosis is changed to Bipolar II Disorder and Cyclothymic Disorder.

   d. Typically, the age of onset is middle adulthood.

   e. In community-based studies, this disorder occurs equally in men and women.

28. All of the following statements regarding the application of the specifiers of Atypical Features to a Mood Disorder are true **EXCEPT**:

   a. Such individuals have little concern about external circumstances or others' opinions of them.

   b. Hypersomnia is an Atypical Feature.

   c. Increased appetite or weight gain is an Atypical Feature.

   d. Affected individuals may complain of feeling heavy or weighted down, especially in the legs and arms—the so-called "leaden paralysis."

   e. Atypical features are more common in women and in younger persons.

29. All of the following statements about the Seasonal Pattern specifier for the Mood Disorders are true **EXCEPT**:

   a. This specifier does not apply to situations better explained by seasonal psychosocial stressors.

   b. Older persons are at higher risk for winter depressive episodes.

   c. Women make up the majority of persons with this disorder.

   d. To be applied to a given case, the pattern of onset and remission must have occurred over the past two years.

   e. Major Depressive Episodes that occur with a seasonal pattern are often characterized by low energy, increased sleep, increased weight, and a craving for carbohydrates.

30. All of the following statements regarding the DSM-IV diagnosis of Panic Attack are true **EXCEPT**:

   a. The Panic Attack is a discrete period that is characterized by intense fear and somatic and/or cognitive symptoms.

   b. Unexpected (uncued) Panic Attacks are without a situational trigger and must be present to diagnose a Panic Disorder.

   c. Situationally bound (cued) Panic Attacks are usually associated with Social or Specific Phobias.

   d. Individuals may experience a limited symptom Panic Attack that meets all the criteria except that it has fewer than 4 of the 13 cognitive/somatic symptoms in DSM-IV.

   e. An exclusive relationship exists between the type of Panic Attack and specific Anxiety Disorders.

31. All of the following statements regarding Panic Disorder are true **EXCEPT**:

   a. DSM-IV requires two unexpected Panic Attacks followed by at least one month of concern about having another attack, or the consequence of having an attack,

or changed behavior due to these attacks.

   b. Many individuals with Panic Disorder have unfocused anxiety unrelated to their Panic Attacks.

   c. Many individuals with Panic Disorder fear a catastrophic outcome from a fairly routine occurrence (e.g., a headache indicates a brain tumor).

   d. Major Depressive Disorder precedes the onset of Panic Disorder in one third of cases.

   e. There is a bimodal distribution of age of onset, with one peak in the mid-30s and a smaller one in the mid-60s.

32. All of the following statements regarding Specific Phobia are true **EXCEPT**:

   a. Having a Specific Phobia from one subtype increases the likelihood of developing another Specific Phobia of a different subtype.

   b. According to DSM-IV, a person expressing an intense fear of snakes, but living in a setting devoid of snakes, having no restrictions due to the fear of snakes, and having no distress about fearing snakes would not have a diagnosis of Specific Phobia.

   c. Adults with this disorder recognize that their fear is excessive and unreasonable.

   d. The frequency in adult clinical setting from most to least frequent is: Situational Type, Natural Environment Type, Blood-Infection-Injury Type, and Animal. Type.

   e. Animal Type and Natural Environment Type frequently have origins in childhood.

33. All of the following statements about Social Phobia are true **EXCEPT**:

   a. The essential feature is a marked and persistent fear of social or performance situations in which embarrassment may occur.

   b. Persons with this diagnosis do not experience anticipatory anxiety about feared events in the future.

   c. Common features associated with this disorder include low self-esteem, underachievement, and a poor social support network.

   d. Adult patients with this disorder frequently have a childhood history of shyness and timidity.

   e. In clinical studies, this diagnosis is equally diagnosed in men and women, or is more common in men.

34. All of the following statements concerning Obsessive-Compulsive Disorder are true **EXCEPT**:

   a. Men with this disorder have an earlier age of onset than do women.

   b. The majority of affected individuals have an insidious onset and a waxing and waning course.

   c. The most common obsessions involve repeated thoughts about contamination, doubts, a need for a particular order of things, and aggressive impulses.

   d. Many patients experience intense anxiety following a compulsive act.

e. The concordance rate for this disorder is higher in monozygotic twins than in dizygotic twins.

35. All of the following statements about Posttraumatic Stress Disorder are true **EXCEPT**:

a. The DSM-IV criteria exclude such events as being diagnosed with a life-threatening illness.

b. Individuals with this disorder typically avoid stimuli associated with the trauma.

c. The affected person's response to the trauma must involve intense fear, helplessness, or horror.

d. Affected persons may reexperience the traumatic event through intrusive recollections or dreams.

e. Onset of symptoms can be delayed for months after the traumatic event.

36. All of the following statements about Generalized Anxiety Disorder are true **EXCEPT**:

a. Affected individuals experience excessive anxiety and worry about a number of events or activities more days than not over a 6-month period.

b. Depressive symptoms are common in affected individuals.

c. During the course of the disorder, the focus of worry remains fixed and unchanging.

d. Frequently, affected individuals complain of poor sleep muscle tension and fatigue.

e. Affected individuals often do not experience their anxiety and worry as excessive.

37. All of the following statements regarding the DSM-IV diagnosis of Substance-Induced Anxiety Disorder are true **EXCEPT**:

a. Heavy metals and hydrocarbons may produce this disorder.

b. This diagnosis is used instead of a diagnosis of Substance Intoxication or Substance Withdrawal only when the anxiety symptoms are judged to be in excess of those usually judged to be associated with Substance Intoxication Withdrawal.

c. Phobic behavior is the most frequently observed anxiety phenomenon in this disorder.

d. This disorder does not occur exclusively during the course of a delirium.

38. All of the following are required for a diagnosis of Somatization Disorder **EXCEPT**:

a. The somatic complaints must begin before age 45.

b. There must be a history of pain in at least four different sites.

c. There must be a history of at least two gastrointestinal complaints other than pain.

d. There must be a history of at least one reproductive or sexual symptom other than pain.

e. There must be a history of at least one symptom suggestive of a neurological condition.

39. All of the following statements about Conversion Disorder are true **EXCEPT**:

a. Conversion symptoms frequently involve voluntary sensory or muscle modalities.

b. Conversion symptoms do not conform to known anatomical or physiological mechanisms.

c. Many individuals with Conversion Disorder have a current or prior neurological condition.

d. A conversion "seizure" will follow a set pattern in the affected individual and not vary from one seizure to another.

e. DSM-IV requires that psychological factors be associated with the onset or exacerbation of the conversion symptoms.

40. All of the following statements regarding Conversion Disorder are true **EXCEPT**:

a. Conversion Disorders are more common in rural areas, lower socioeconomic status, and developing regions.

b. Conversion Disorders in children under the age of 10 are usually limited to genitourinary problems.

c. The form of conversion symptoms reflects local and cultural ideas about acceptable and credible ways to express distress.

d. Conversion Disorder rarely has a new onset after the age of 35.

e. Women are more frequently affected than are men, and symptoms are more common on the left side of the body than on the right in affected women.

41. All of the following statements are true of Hypochondriasis **EXCEPT**:

a. Affected individuals are preoccupied with having a serious disease based on a misinterpretation of bodily signs and symptoms.

b. The belief that one has a disease is often of delusional intensity.

c. Repeated negative physical examinations and laboratory findings do not reassure the affected individual about the absence of physical disease.

d. Serious illness in childhood and past experience of a disease in a family member may predispose the individual to this disorder.

e. The disorder is equally common in males and females and has a usual age of onset in early adulthood.

42. All of the following statements about Factitious Disorder are correct **EXCEPT**:

a. Complaints of pain and requests for pain medication are common in this patient population.

b. Patients with this disorder present their complaints with dramatic flair but are very vague and inconsistent when questioned in detail.

c. In Factitious Disorder with Predominantly Psychological Signs and Symptoms, approximate answers may be given.

d. Possible predisposing factors may be extensive medical treatment and hospitalization during childhood and adolescence.

e. Incentives for the behavior exhibited by these individuals include economic gain and freedom from legal responsibility.

43. All of the following statements regarding types of amnesia are true EXCEPT:

a. Localized Amnesia refers to amnesias related to specific sites where a traumatic or stressful event occurred.

b. Selective Amnesia refers to the inability to recall some of the events that occurred during a certain span of time.

c. Generalized Amnesia is a rare condition resulting in the inability to recall events subsequent to a specific time up to and including the present.

d. Systematized Amnesia is the loss of memory for specific categories of information.

e. The most common types of Amnesia are localized and elective.

44. Which of the following statements is true of Dissociative Fugue?

a. The essential feature is sudden, unexpected travel away from home with an inability to recall some or all of one's past.

b. If a new identity is assumed during a fugue, it is usually of a quieter, more withdrawn nature than was the nonfugue personality.

c. During a fugue, the affected individual appears to be free of psychopathology.

d. When an affected individual returns to a prefugue state, no memory of events taking place during the fugue is retained.

e. Recovery is usually rapid.

45. All of the following statements regarding Dissociative Identity Disorder are true EXCEPT:

a. Transition between identities is often triggered by psychosocial stress.

b. Each personality state is experienced as if it has a distinct personality, history, self-image, and identity.

c. The primary identity that carries the individual's given name is usually aggressive, hostile, and controlling.

d. This disorder represents a failure to integrate various aspects of memory, identity, and consciousness.

e. Most frequently, there are 10 or fewer identities in affected individuals.

46. All of the following statements regarding Depersonalization Disorder are true EXCEPT:

a. Feelings of detachment or estrangement from one's self are the defining characteristics of this disorder.

b. Depersonalization is a common experience occurring both in many mental disorders and in individuals free of mental disorders.

c. During the depersonalization episode the affected individual's reality testing is impaired or lost.

d. Individuals with Depersonalization Disorder may be easily hypnotized and have a high dissociative capacity.

e. Approximately half of adults may have experienced brief episodes of depersonalization, usually precipitated by severe stress.

47. All of the following statements regarding Hypoactive Sexual Desire Disorder are true EXCEPT:

a. Individuals with this disorder have a deficiency or absence of sexual fantasies or desire for sexual activity.

b. By definition, the low sex drive is global and affects all aspects of sexual expression.

c. Affected individuals do not initiate sexual activity.

d. Most frequently, this disorder develops in adulthood in response to stress or interpersonal difficulties after a period of normal sexual interest.

e. The clinician should assess both partners to develop a more comprehensive picture of the couple's sexual drives, both as individuals and as a couple.

48. All of the following statements about Orgasmic Disorder are true EXCEPT:

a. Males with the diagnosis of Male Orgasmic Disorder do not attain orgasm.

b. Females with this disorder tend to have had a lifelong course of anorgasmia.

c. In males, age should be taken into account before making the diagnosis.

d. No association has been found between specific patterns of personality traits or psychopathology and orgasmic dysfunction in females.

e. Female Orgasmic Disorder is more prevalent in younger women because orgasmic capacity in females increases with age.

49. All of the following statements regarding the DSM-IV diagnosis of Premature Ejaculation are true EXCEPT:

a. Such factors as age, novelty of situation, and frequency of sexual activity are important in evaluating a patient suspected of having this disorder.

b. Most men with this disorder cannot delay orgasm even when masturbating.

c. The essential feature is the persistent onset of orgasm and ejaculation with minimal stimulation before the patient desires it.

d. The clinician should evaluate the partners' estimate of the duration of time from the beginning of sexual activity to ejaculation.

e. Typically, young males with little sexual experience may present with this disorder.

50. In the DSM-IV, which of the following is not seen in a Manic Episode?

a. Persistent explosive or irritable mood

b. Abnormal mood lasting at least a week

c. Poor self-esteem

d. Flight of ideas

51. All of the following statements about Anorexia Nervosa are true **EXCEPT**:

a. Individuals with this disorder have an altered perception of hunger.

b. Individuals with this disorder refuse to maintain a normal body weight.

c. Individuals with this disorder are intensely afraid of gaining weight.

d. Individuals with this disorder have a significant distortion of the shape or size of the body.

e. Postmenarcheal females with this disorder are amenorrheic.

52. All of the following statements about Anorexia Nervosa are true **EXCEPT**:

a. Individuals with this diagnosis rarely complain of weight loss.

b. Some individuals may use restricting food or food types as a weight-control mechanism, others may use a binge–purge method, and some use both methods.

c. Individuals with this diagnosis avoid food-related activities such as cooking and recipe collecting.

d. This disorder tends to be far more prevalent in industrialized countries.

e. The onset of the disorder rarely occurs before puberty and after the age of 40.

53. All of the following statements are true of Bulimia Nervosa **EXCEPT**:

a. Individuals with this diagnosis place excessive emphasis on body shape and weight in their self-evaluations.

b. Individuals with this disorder are typically underweight.

c. Depressive and anxious symptoms may be present in individuals with this disorder.

d. This disorder is more common in industrialized countries.

e. The prevalence rate is about 1–3% in adolescent and young adult females.

54. All of the following statements are true of normal sleep **EXCEPT**:

a. Rapid-eye-movement (REM) sleep is cyclical and occurs at 80–100-minute intervals.

b. There are five distinct stages of sleep: REM sleep and stages 1–4.

c. Most REM sleep occurs in the first one third of sleep.

d. Fifty percent of total sleep time is spent in stage 2 sleep.

e. Sleep continuity and depth deteriorate with age.

55. All of the following statements regarding Primary Insomnia are true **EXCEPT**:

a. Most cases have a sudden onset during a time of stress.

b. The typical course of illness is a period of progressive sleep difficulties, followed by a chronic phase of sleep disturbance.

c. This diagnosis is rarely made before young adulthood.

d. Sleep laboratory studies support the complaints about poor sleep reported by elderly women.

e. In clinics specializing in sleep disorders, 15–25% of the patients will be diagnosed with Primary Insomnia.

56. Which one of the following statements about the diagnosis of Primary Hypersomnia is true?

a. The duration of the sleep episode is greater than 16 hours followed by easy arousal and normal daytime alertness.

b. The sleep architecture is abnormal, with prolonged periods of stage 3 and stage 4 sleep.

c. Daytime naps tend to be long (greater than one hour), are experienced as unrefreshing, and are not helpful in combating daytime sleepiness.

d. Daytime naps are often abrupt in onset and occur without warning.

e. Less than 1% of patients in sleep disorder clinics have this diagnosis.

57. All of the following statements concerning Narcolepsy are true **EXCEPT**:

a. The sleep attacks of Narcolepsy are irresistible, last 10–20 minutes, and are refreshing for the individual.

b. Seventy percent of patients experience cataplexy, the sudden loss of muscle tone brought on by intense emotion.

c. Some 30% to 50% of patients experience sleep paralysis as a part of the narcoleptic syndrome.

d. Persons with untreated Narcolepsy average 10–15 sleep attacks a day.

e. Individuals with Narcolepsy experience intensely vivid dreamlike hallucinations at sleep emergence or at sleep onset.

58. All of the following statements about the DSM-IV diagnosis of Breathing Related Sleep Disorder are true **EXCEPT**:

a. Excessive sleepiness is the most common presenting complaint.

b. The individual will have frequent awakenings or arousals during the night as a part of an attempt to breathe normally.

c. Daytime naps in these individuals tend to be unrefreshing and to be accompanied by a dull headache.

d. Severe dryness of the mouth is common.

e. Sleep studies of persons with this disorder show that they have less body movement during sleep than do normal sleepers.

59. All of the following statements about Circadian Rhythm Sleep Disorder are true **EXCEPT**:

a. Rotating-shift schedules are the most disruptive to

sleep patterns because they force sleep and wakefulness into aberrant circadian positions and prevent any consistent adjustment.

b. The central aspect of this disorder is the mismatch of the external demands for activity at a given time, and these demands conflict with the person's intrinsic circadian rhythm.

c. In the Delayed Sleep Phase Type of this disorder, the individual will go to bed later on the weekends and on vacation.

d. Jet Lag and Shift Work Types are more common in individuals who are "night owls."

e. Delayed Sleep Phase Type is more common in individuals who have characteristics of Schizoid, Avoidant, and Schizotypal personalities.

60. All of the following statements about the DSM-IV diagnosis of Nightmare Disorder are true **EXCEPT**:

a. The essential feature is the repeated occurrence of frightening dreams that lead to sleep disruption.

b. The individual is groggy and only partially awake following a nightmare event that results in an awakening.

c. The nightmares typically occur in lengthy, involved dream sequences that are anxiety provoking or are terrifying.

d. Individuals with this disorder typically remember the dream sequence in detail.

e. Nightmares typically occur with greater frequency in the latter half of the sleep cycle since that is when most REM sleep occurs.

61. Sleep Terror Disorder is characterized by all of the following **EXCEPT**:

a. A typical episode involves the person's abruptly sitting up and screaming or crying but having no recollection of a coherent dream.

b. The individual is usually unresponsive to those who seek to awaken or comfort him or her.

c. The individual is usually amnestic for the event the next day.

d. Sleep Terror Disorder typically occurs during REM sleep.

e. Sleep Terror Disorder typically begins in children age 12 and resolves spontaneously in adolescence.

62. All of the following statements regarding the diagnosis Intermittent Explosive Disorder are true **EXCEPT**:

a. The disorder apparently is rare.

b. The episodes of aggressiveness are the only times the individual expresses aggression.

c. Typical of the Impulse Control Disorder, the patient experiences tension or arousal before an episode and a sense of relief following the episode.

d. The essential feature of the diagnosis is the occurrence of discrete episodes of failure to resist aggressive impulses.

e. The degree of aggression expressed during an episode

is grossly out of proportion to any provocation preceding it.

63. All of the following statements about Pyromania are true **EXCEPT**:

a. Although 40% of all arson arrests are of persons under the age of 18, this a rare disorder in childhood.

b. Individuals with this disorder may make extensive plans for starting fires, in sharp contrast to those with other Impulse Control Disorders, who most often act without planning.

c. Individuals with this disorder are frequently preoccupied with fire and fire-related activities.

d. Individuals with this disorder often set fires in response to a delusion or a hallucination.

e. By definition, the fire-setting behavior is not for monetary gain, to express political conviction, or to conceal criminal activity.

64. Trichotillomania:

a. Is the recurrent pulling out of one's own hair without noticeable hair loss.

b. Does not have pain routinely associated with the hair pulling.

c. Involves tension preceding the act of hair pulling, but not with attempts to resist the urge to pull the hair.

d. Is more common among females in both child and adult populations.

e. Is limited to pulling hair from one's own body and not from other persons or from objects.

65. All of the following statements about Adjustment Disorder are true **EXCEPT**:

a. The diagnosis of Adjustment Disorder does not apply when the symptoms represent Bereavement.

b. The essential feature is the development of clinically significant emotional or behavioral problems in response to an identifiable psychosocial stressor.

c. The symptoms must develop within one month of the psychosocial stressors.

d. The Adjustment Disorder must resolve within 6 months of its onset.

e. A decreased performance in school or at work is a frequently associated feature of Adjustment Disorder.

66. All of the following statements are true **EXCEPT**:

a. When evaluating an individual for a Personality Disorder, ethnic, social, and cultural factors must be considered.

b. To diagnose a Personality Disorder in a person under the age of 18, the symptoms must have been present for at least one year, except in the diagnosis of Antisocial Personality Disorder.

c. The development of personality changes in middle adulthood or later should be thoroughly evaluated for possible medical causes.

d. Maladaptive personality traits that do not meet the

threshold for a Personality Disorder can be coded on Axis II.

e. External events, such as job loss or divorce, have little effect on the emergence of Personality Disorders.

67. All of the following statements about the Paranoid Personality Disorder are true **EXCEPT**:

   a. Alcohol and other Substance Abuse or Dependence frequently occur in association with this disorder.
   b. Individuals may exhibit thinly hidden unrealistic grandiose fantasies about power and rank.
   c. In response to stress, these individuals may experience brief episodes of psychosis, lasting minutes to hours.
   d. Individuals with this diagnosis tend to avoid group activities since they are so distrustful of others.
   e. In some cases, this diagnosis may be the antecedent of Delusional Disorder or of Schizophrenia.

68. All of the following statements about Schizotypal Personality Disorder are true **EXCEPT**:

   a. Paranoid ideation is not a part of the clinical picture in this disorder.
   b. The speech of these individuals may be vague or digressive, but it is not incoherent and it lacks the characteristics of derailment.
   c. Individuals with this disorder often seek treatment for their dysphoric affects.
   d. Cognitive and perceptual disturbances are the hallmarks of this disorder.
   e. When admitted to a clinical setting, 30–50% of individuals with this diagnosis will have a concurrent diagnosis of Major Depressive Disorder.

69. All the following statements about Antisocial Personality Disorder are true **EXCEPT**:

   a. The essential feature of this disorder is a pervasive pattern of disregard for, and violation of, the rights of others.
   b. To be given this diagnosis, a person must be at least 18 years old, but have had a history of some symptoms before the age of 15.
   c. Individuals with this disorder are calculating and cautious in their manipulation of other and do not display impulsivity or volatility as part of the clinical picture.
   d. Consistent and extreme irresponsibility is highly characteristic of the disorder.
   e. Lack of empathy, inflated self-appraisal, and superficial charm are features commonly associated with individuals with this disorder.

70. All of the following statements regarding the diagnosis of Borderline Personality Disorder are true **EXCEPT**:

   a. Suicide attempts are very common in this population with 8–10% of individuals with the diagnosis completing suicide.
   b. Individuals in this population may have feelings of emptiness, are easily bored, and may constantly seek something to do.
   c. The emotional volatility of the individual with this diagnosis is linked to an intense fear of separation.
   d. Seventy-five percent of individuals with this diagnosis are female.
   e. Increasing age is usually associated with a greater severity of symptoms in individuals with this diagnosis.

71. All of the following statements about Histrionic Personality Disorder are true **EXCEPT**:

   a. These individuals have a high degree of suggestibility and are easily swayed by the opinions of others.
   b. The behavioral expression of the person with Histrionic Personality Disorder is not influenced by sex role stereotypes.
   c. The individuals are intolerant of situations requiring delayed gratification.
   d. Impressionistic and impressive speech are characteristics of the disorder.
   e. The prevalence is about 2–3% in the general population.

72. All of the following statements are true of Narcissistic Personality Disorder **EXCEPT**:

   a. Persons with the disorder believe that they are special, unique, and superior, and thus the opinions that others have of them are irrelevant to them.
   b. These individuals have a pervasive pattern of grandiosity and lack of empathy that begins in early adulthood.
   c. These individuals are consumed by their own feelings and fail to recognize that others also have feelings and needs.
   d. These individuals expect others to be totally concerned about their welfare.
   e. Vocational functioning may be very low since these individuals will not risk defeat in competitive situations.

73. All of the following are characteristics of Dependent Personality Disorder **EXCEPT**:

   a. Persons with this disorder allow others to take the initiative and to assume responsibility for most areas of their lives.
   b. They lack the self-confidence to carry out tasks, always believing that they need the help of others.
   c. These individuals have strong needs for emotional support and nurturance and will disagree vigorously with those who refuse to meet their demands for this level of emotional support.
   d. This disorder is among the Personality Disorders most frequently diagnosed in mental health clinics.
   e. These individuals will often tolerate physical, emotional, or sexual abuse to ensure that they receive their perceived emotional nurturance.

74. All of the following statements are true **EXCEPT**:

    a. The major pathway implicated in the genesis of Delirium is the dorsal tegmental pathway.

    b. Delirium associated with alcohol had been associated with the locus ceruleus and its noradrenergic neurons.

    c. The major transmitter believed to be involved with Delirium is serotonin.

    d. Medications are common causes of Delirium.

    e. The reticular activating formation is believed to be involved in delirium because it is involved in arousal and attention, two functions that are impaired with Delirium.

75. All of the following statements are true **EXCEPT**:

    a. Transient ischemic attacks are brief episodes of focal neurological dysfunction lasting less than 24 hours and having no pathological alteration of parenchymal tissue.

    b. Patients with pseudodementia complain more of cognitive loss than do patients with an organic basis for their dementia.

    c. Ninety percent of patient with Dementia of the Alzheimers's Type experience their first symptom between the ages of 65 and 70.

    d. Dementia due to HIV Disease is associated with significant motor impairment, as well as cognitive impairment.

    e. Minor memory problems are associated with the aging process.

76. All of the following statements are true **EXCEPT**:

    a. Approximately 40% of the population have used an illicit drug at some point in their lives.

    b. The most commonly used illicit drug is cocaine or some form of cocaine (e.g., crack cocaine).

    c. Eighty-five percent of the population have used alcohol at some point in their lives.

    d. Seventy-five percent of the population have smoked cigarettes at some point in their lives.

    e. Of the population age 12 and older, 33% have used cannabis (marijuana) at some point in their lifetimes.

77. Cell membranes receptors have been identified for most substances with the exception of:

    a. Opiates

    b. Benzodiazepines

    c. Cocaine

    d. Alcohol

    e. LSD

78. All of the following statements regarding anabolic steroids are true **EXCEPT**:

    a. About half of the users of these drugs begin such use before the age of 16.

    b. Psychiatric symptoms associated with the use of these drugs include irritability, euphoria, and hyperactivity.

    c. Depression may occur during periods when steroids are not being used.

    d. Episodes of violence during steroid use occur exclusively in individuals who have a history of violence or of sociopathy.

    e. Anabolic steroids are schedule III drugs.

79. Regarding the physiological effects of alcohol, which of the following statements is false?

    a. The intoxicating effects of alcohol are as great when the blood alcohol level is falling as when the blood alcohol level is rising.

    b. The average rate of oxidation of alcohol by the liver is about 15 mg/dl/hr, approximately the amount of alcohol contained in a moderate-sized drink.

    c. Ninety percent of alcohol is metabolized by the liver at a constant rate and the remainder is excreted unchanged by the lungs and the kidneys.

    d. Drinking alcohol on an empty stomach enhances its absorption.

    e. Most alcohol consumed is absorbed by the small intestine.

80. All of the following statements about alcohol withdrawal seizures are true **EXCEPT**:

    a. These seizures are generally stereotypic and generalized and tonic-clonic in type.

    b. Alcohol withdrawal seizures usually occur singly and do not occur more than once in a withdrawal situation.

    c. Status epilepticus is rare in alcohol withdrawal.

    d. Other causes of seizures, such as head trauma, must be evaluated.

    e. Anticonvulsants are not indicated in the management of alcohol withdrawal seizures.

81. All of the following statements regarding Delirium Tremors (DTs) are true **EXCEPT**:

    a. Untreated, DTs has a mortality rate of 20%, usually as a result of an underlying medical condition.

    b. DTs typically begins on the third hospital day.

    c. Perceptual problems, such as tactile and visual hallucinations, are common.

    d. Benzodiazepines are useful in the treatment of the withdrawal symptoms.

    e. Signs of sympathetic hypoactivity, such as lethargy, bradycardia, and hypotension, are common in this clinical picture.

82. All of the following statements about alcohol-related blackouts are true **EXCEPT**:

    a. During a blackout, intellectual capabilities are preserved.

    b. Blackouts are similar to transient global amnesia in that they are discrete periods of antegrade amnesia.

    c. During a blackout, all spheres of memory—remote, recent, and immediate—are impaired.

    d. Patients with blackouts experience much distress when their inappropriate actions during blackouts are reported to them.

e. Alcohol blocks the consolidation of recent memories into remote memories.

83. All the following statements are true **EXCEPT**:

   a. Amphetamines act by causing the release of dopamine and norepinephrine in the central nervous system.
   b. The effects of dopamine and norepinephrine release caused by the amphetamines are particularly prominent in the ventral tegmental area to the cortex and the limbic areas.
   c. The designer amphetamines (for example, MDMA, MDEA, MMDA, and DOM) also cause the release of serotonin, the neurotransmitter implicated in hallucinatory drugs.
   d. Fluoxetine and MDMA have synergistic effects.
   e. All amphetamines are rapidly absorbed after oral administration.

84. All the following statements about caffeine are true **EXCEPT**:

   a. A cup of coffee contains about 100–150 mg of caffeine.
   b. The average adult in the Untied States consumes about 200 mg of caffeine a day and 20–30% consume more than 500 mg.
   c. Caffeine is a methylxanthine and is more potent than the other commonly used xanthine, theophylline.
   d. Caffeine does not possess the traits commonly associated with drugs of abuse.
   e. The primary mechanism of action for caffeine is as an antagonist for adenosine receptors.

85. All of the following statements about cannabis (marijuana) are true **EXCEPT**:

   a. The drug is predominantly used by adolescents and young adults.
   b. A specific receptor for cannabis has been identified.
   c. Most studies demonstrate that animals will self-administer cannabis, as is typical of drugs of abuse.
   d. Withdrawal symptoms associated with chronic cannabis use include modest increases in irritability, restlessness, insomnia, and anorexia, and mild nausea.
   e. Common physical findings associated with cannabis intoxication include red eyes, mild tachycardia, increased appetite, and dry mouth.

86. Adverse effects associated with cocaine use include all of the following **EXCEPT**:

   a. Seizures
   b. Myocardial infarction
   c. Psychomotor retardation
   d. Inflammation and mucosal damage to the nasal passages
   e. Nonhemorrhagic cerebral infarction

87. Issues commonly encountered in the treatment of cocaine abusers include all of the following **EXCEPT**:

   a. Resistance to entering a treatment program.
   b. Intense craving for cocaine during the initial phase of withdrawal.
   c. The need for hospitalization in the early phases to prevent relapse.
   d. Frequent and random urine drug screens, which are almost always necessary to ensure the patient's continued abstinence.
   e. All of the above.

88. Correct statements about the use of hallucinogens in the United States include all of the following **EXCEPT**:

   a. Less than 10% of the U.S. population report use of a hallucinogen at anytime during their lives.
   b. The most common demographic profile of a hallucinogen user is an African-American male living in the western United States who is between the age of 15 and 35.
   c. Hallucinogen use is associated with less mortality and morbidity than are other substances.
   d. Rates of lifetime use by older adults have steadily increased from 1974 to the present.
   e. Only 1% of emergency room visits are related to hallucinogen use.

89. All of the following statements about inhalant use are true **EXCEPT**:

   a. Most of the inhalants are metabolized in the liver, with a small percentage being excreted by the lungs.
   b. Concurrent use of alcohol with the inhalants will decrease the intoxicating effects of the inhalant.
   c. The typical experiences associated with inhalant use are euphoria, excitement, and pleasant floating sensations.
   d. Usually an individual uses inhalants for only a short time during his or her life.
   e. Organic solvents in combination with heavy metals may result in brain atrophy, temporal lobe epilepsy, and decreased intelligence.

90. All of the following statements about tobacco use and nicotine are true **EXCEPT**:

   a. Tobacco use in psychiatric patients is high, with 50% of outpatients, 70% of patients with Bipolar Disorder, and 90% of patients with Schizophrenia smoking.
   b. The rate of smoking in the general population is about 27%.
   c. Nicotine may exert its addictive qualities by stimulating the dopaminergic pathways projecting from the ventral tegmental area to the cortex and the limbic system.
   d. Nicotine is a highly addicting, but relatively innocuous substance with no known overdose.
   e. Sixty percent of the direct health care costs in the United States go to treat tobacco-related illnesses, or about $1 billion a day.

91. All of the following statements are true **EXCEPT**:

    a. Specific opiate receptors are in the central nervous system.
    b. The addictive qualities of the opiates may be mediated by dopaminergic pathways of the ventral tegmental area.
    c. Opiates have effects on both the dopaminergic and norepinephrine systems.
    d. Heroin is more potent and lipid soluble than is morphine.
    e. Codeine is rapidly absorbed by the gastrointestinal tract and is converted to heroin.

92. All of the following statements about persons addicted to opioids and addiction are true **EXCEPT**:

    a. Withdrawal symptoms from morphine or heroin begin six to eight hours after the last dose.
    b. Withdrawal symptoms from opiates include diarrhea, musculoskeletal pain, rhinorrhea, lacrimation, and yawning.
    c. Tolerance to the opioids develops rapidly.
    d. Death from an opioid overdose is almost always due to cardiac arrest.
    e. Opiate antagonists produce an almost immediate withdrawal syndrome after their infusion.

93. All of the following statements about phencyclidine (PCP) are true **EXCEPT**:

    a. The anesthetic ketamine, used in humans, is related to PCP and is subject to abuse.
    b. The primary pharmacodynamic activity of PCP is the binding to NMDA receptors.
    c. PCP stimulates the dopaminergic pathways of the ventral tegmental area.
    d. Like most drugs of abuse, PCP produces both tolerance and physical dependence.
    e. The highest rate of PCP use in the United States is in the Washington D.C. area.

94. Which of the following statements regarding the treatment of a patient who has ingested PCP is correct?

    a. Benzodiazepines should be avoided for the management of the acute agitation caused by PCP ingestion.
    b. Severe hypotension may complicate the clinical management of these patients.
    c. Talking the patient down is not effective in these patients.
    d. Four-point restraints should be routinely used to prevent injury to the patient or to others.
    e. Alkalization of the urine will speed excretion of the PCP.

95. Sudden death is most common in the withdrawal syndrome of which of the following drugs?

    a. Alcohol
    b. Barbiturates
    c. Benzodiazepines
    d. Opiates
    e. Hallucinogens

96. Which of the following statements is false?

    a. In the United States, persons with Schizophrenia more often were born in the months of January to April.
    b. Schizophrenic patients who smoke have a greater likelihood of developing drug-induced parkinsonism.
    c. Schizophrenic persons have greater mortality rate from both accidents and natural causes than do members of the general population.
    d. Suicide is a common cause of death among schizophrenic patients.
    e. The fertility rate for schizophrenic persons is close to that of the general population.

97. Which of the following statements is false?

    a. The dopaminergic hypothesis of Schizophrenia posits that patients with the disorder have excessive dopaminergic activity.
    b. All effective antipsychotic medications have a direct correlation between their ability to block dopamine type 2 receptors and their potency and efficacy.
    c. Studies indicate a positive correlation between the plasma concentration of homovanillic acid, the severity of the psychotic symptoms, and the response to antipsychotic medications.
    d. Serotonin activity has been implicated in the impulsive and suicidal behavior of schizophrenic patients.
    e. Computerized axial tomography of the brains of schizophrenic patients consistently demonstrate enlargement of the lateral and third ventricles, with some reduction in brain volume.

98. All of the following statements regarding perceptual disturbances are true **EXCEPT**:

    a. The difference between an illusion and a hallucination is that the illusions are based on real stimuli.
    b. Olfactory and gustatory hallucinations are common in the schizophrenic population.
    c. Hearing two or more voices offering running, usually negative, commentary on the patient's behavior is a quite common experience among schizophrenic individuals.
    d. A cenesthetic hallucination is an unfounded sensation of an altered body state in a body organ.

99. Risk factors for suicide in a schizophrenic individual include all of the following **EXCEPT**:

    a. Being female
    b. Having a college education
    c. Being young
    d. Experiencing a change in the course of an illness
    e. Living alone

100. All of the following statements about Postpartum Psychosis are true **EXCEPT**:

a. Most of the women with this disorder have just had their first child.

b. Most of the women with this disorder do not require hospitalization and can be treated as outpatients so as not to disrupt the bonding of mother and child.

c. Fifty percent of women with this disorder have nonpsychiatric perinatal complications.

d. Relatives of persons with Postpartum Psychosis have an incidence of Mood Disorder that is similar to that of relatives or persons with Mood Disorders.

e. Treatment with an antidepressant and lithium may be the treatment of choice.

101. Correct statements about the treatment of Delusional Disorder include all of the following **EXCEPT**:

a. Reasons to consider hospitalization for these patients include violent impulses, the need for medical and neurological evaluation, and social and occupational dysfunction.

b. Most patients with this disorder can be treated as outpatients.

c. A professional, well-defined therapeutic stance may set the correct tone for any psychotherapy with these patients.

d. The projection used as a defense mechanism must be directly confronted by the therapist.

e. In patients who respond to antipsychotics, maintenance doses are usually low.

102–105. Match the following with the description.

a. Amok
b. Cotard's syndrome
c. Capgras's syndrome
d. Autoscopic psychosis

102. A visual hallucination of all or part of one's body.

103. Sudden unprovoked outburst of wild rage.

104. Delusion that persons close to one have been replaced by impostors.

105. The world beyond the patient is reduced to nothingness in this disorder.

**DIRECTIONS: For questions 106 through 174, one or more of the alternatives may be correct. After deciding which of the alternatives are correct, record your answer according to the following key.**

**A.** Alternatives 1, 2, and 3 are correct.
**B.** Alternatives 1 and 3 are correct.
**C.** Alternatives 2 and 4 are correct.
**D.** Alternative 4 only is correct.
**E.** All four alternatives are correct.

106. Which of the following statements about Gender Identity Disorder is/are true?

1. In order to make this diagnosis, there must be a strong and persistent cross-gender identification that is the desire to be, or the insistence that one is, of the other sex.

2. Children with this disorder generally are homosexual as adults.

3. The individual with this disorder experiences persistent discomfort in assigned sex role or a sense of inappropriateness in the assigned sex role.

4. While these affected individuals experience intense emotional distress, they usually will adhere to the normative behavior of their assigned sex rather than risk parental or societal disapproval.

107. Which of the following statements is/are true of Bulimia Nervosa?

1. Snacking continuously during the day qualifies as a binge.

2. A binge refers to the consumption of an amount of food that is definitely larger than what an individual would ordinarily consume during a discrete period of time.

3. Binges usually do not have external conditions that act as triggers but occur spontaneously.

4. The most common mechanism for compensating for overeating is purging, (i.e., self-induced vomiting).

108. Which of the following statements regarding the diagnosis of Primary Insomnia is/are true?

1. Most often, individuals with the diagnosis report difficulty in falling asleep or difficulty in maintaining sleep.

2. Occasionally, individuals with this diagnosis will complain only of nonrestorative sleep.

3. Many individuals with this diagnosis have a lifelong history of poor sleep.

4. Complaints of insomnia are more prevalent in older persons and in women.

109. Which of the following statements is/are true of the Kleine-Levin syndrome?

1. Males and females are equally affected by this syndrome.

2. Between periods of excessive sleep, clinical manifestations of disinhibition may be manifest.

3. Marked decreases in appetite with significant weight loss may occur.

4. Hypersexuality marked by inappropriate sexual advances may also appear during the course of illness.

110. Which of the following statements about Narcolepsy is/are true?

1. Approximately 25–50% of first-degree biological relatives of individuals with Narcolepsy have disorders characterized by excessive sleepiness.

2. The excessive sleepiness of Narcolepsy is stable over time.
3. Daytime sleepiness is almost always the first symptom of Narcolepsy.
4. The male-to-female ratio for this disorder is 2:1.

111. Which of the following statements about obstructive sleep apnea syndrome is/are correct?

1. This is the least common type of sleep apnea.
2. Breathing cessation is for ten seconds or less and is not associated with cyanosis.
3. Most affected individuals are aware of their sleep problems before bed partners are.
4. Affected individuals snore loudly enough to disturb the sleep of bed partners.

112. Which of the following statements is/are correct?

1. Central sleep apnea is associated with episodic cessation of breathing without airway obstruction.
2. Central alveolar hyperventilation syndrome occurs mostly in very overweight people.
3. Central sleep apnea is more common in elderly populations.
4. In adults, the male-to-female ratio of obstructive sleep apnea is 4:1.

113. Which of the following statements about Sleepwalking Disorder is/are true?

1. Injury to the individual during a sleepwalking episode is quite rare.
2. The behaviors exhibited during an episode are usually of low complexity and are routine.
3. Sleepwalking episodes occur during REM sleep.
4. Sleepwalking most commonly occurs for the first time between the ages of 4 and 8.

114. Which of the following statements about Kleptomania is/are true?

1. This is a rare condition, and is more common in females.
2. The individual is aware that the stealing is wrong and senseless.
3. The individual fears arrest or other negative consequences for the stealing.
4. The act of stealing is frequently an expression of anger or rage.

115. Which of the following statements about Pathological Gambling is/are true?

1. Individuals with this disorder are preoccupied with gambling and often seek higher and higher stakes to achieve the desired level of excitement.
2. Approximately one third of all pathological gamblers are female.
3. Pathological Gambling and Alcohol Dependence are both more common in the parents of individuals with the diagnosis of Pathological Gambling than in the general public.
4. Individuals with this diagnosis are often highly competitive, and energetic and are easily bored.

116. Which of the following statements is/are true of Personality Disorders in general?

1. Only when personality traits are inflexible and maladaptive do they constitute a diagnosis of Personality Disorder.
2. The pattern of personality traits is enduring and pervasive over a variety of situations, and evaluation of the individual's long-term functioning is required for diagnosis.
3. The stable pattern of personality traits can be traced back to adolescence or early adulthood.
4. The individual with this diagnosis always experiences the inflexible and maladaptive personality traits as ego dystonic.

117. Which of the following statements about Paranoid Personality Disorders is/are true?

1. Individuals with this disorder have an extreme distrust of strangers, but the people they do trust are trusted completely and without question.
2. Individuals with this disorder are generally easy to get along with in a job setting because they are not forthcoming with personal information and thus are better able to focus on work-related tasks.
3. Although individuals with this disorder are suspicious of those they do not know, jealousy is not a part of the picture.
4. Individuals with this disorder bear grudges and are unwilling to forgive perceived insults or slights.

118. Which of the following statements about Schizoid Personality Disorder is/are true?

1. Individuals with this disorder are excessively sensitive to others' assessments of them and thus withdraw from the world.
2. These individuals have a chronically sad or depressed affect.
3. These individuals may have an especially close relationship with their immediate families, but have little interest in or the ability to develop relationships outside of the family.
4. Schizoid Personality Disorder is an uncommon disorder and may be more common and disabling in males.

119. Which of the following statements about Antisocial Personality Disorder is/are true?

1. Complaints of tension, inability to tolerate boredom, and depressed mood are often associated features.
2. Antisocial Personality Disorder appears to be associated with low socioeconomic status and urban life.
3. The overall prevalence of this disorder in community samples appears to be 3% for males and 1% for females.

4. First-degree biological relatives of these individuals may have a higher incidence of Somatization Disorder.

120. Which of the following statements is/are true of Avoidant Personality Disorder?

1. These individuals avoid interpersonal activities because they are fearful of criticism or rejection.
2. Feelings of inferiority and low self-esteem result in an inhibited life.
3. These individuals have a strong desire for love from and acceptance by others.
4. The avoidant behavior usually begins in early adulthood after normal development during childhood and adolescence.

121. Which of the following statements about Obsessive-Compulsive Personality Disorder is/are true?

1. While they are mercilessly critical of the shortcomings and imperfections of others, they hold up their own selves and behaviors as models of perfection.
2. Rigidity of thinking and inflexibility are hallmarks of this disorder.
3. These individuals are quick to make a decision and will adamantly stand by their decision even when abandoning it would be in their best interest.
4. Individuals with this disorder are miserly and live far below their means.

122. Which of the following statements is/are true?

1. In contrast to the parietal-temporal distribution of pathology in Dementia of the Alzheimer's Type, Dementia due to Pick's Disease is characterized by a preponderance of atrophy in the frontotemporal regions.
2. Neurotransmitters implicated in the pathophysiology of Dementia of the Alzheimer's Type are not epinephrine and acetylcholine.
3. Vascular dementia is more common in men who have hypertension.
4. Binswanger's disease is characterized by multiple small infarctions in the cerebral cortex.

123. Which of the following statements is/are true of Korsakoff's syndrome?

1. This syndrome may be associated with chronic alcoholism.
2. Other medical problems that can result in poor nutrition may produce this syndrome.
3. Confabulation, apathy, and passivity are prominent symptoms of this disorder.
4. Thiamine deficiency is the cause of this syndrome.

124. Psychotherapeutic issues that are prominent in HIV-infected patients include:

1. Health care issues, including specific treatments and medications

2. Terminal care and life support
3. Issues regarding self-esteem and self-blame
4. Issues regarding substance abuse

125. With regard to comorbidity:

1. It is defined as having two or more diagnoses in a single patient.
2. Twenty percent of men and 15% of women with a diagnosis of Substance Abuse or Substance Dependence have an additional psychiatric diagnosis.
3. The most common psychiatric condition with Substance Abuse or Substance Dependence is Antisocial Personality Disorder.
4. In general, the most potent and dangerous substances have the lowest comorbidity rates.

126. Which of the following has/have been implicated in the etiology of Alcohol-Related Disorders?

1. Anxiety fixated at the oral stage of development may be lessened by the intake of alcohol.
2. Individuals with first-degree relatives who have Alcohol-Related Disorders have a greater risk of developing Alcohol-Related Disorders.
3. Certain environments, such as college dorms and military installations, may tolerate and even encourage overuse of alcohol.
4. Familial drinking habits are the most important factor in determining the drinking habits of offspring.

127. Which of the following statements about Wernicke's syndrome is/are true?

1. Untreated, this syndrome may progress to Korsakoff's syndrome.
2. Untreated Korsakoff's syndrome results in Wernicke's syndrome.
3. Wernicke's syndrome causes ataxia, primarily affecting the gait.
4. The eye findings of Wernicke's syndrome are usually unilateral.

128. Which of the following statements about the Fetal Alcohol Syndrome is/are true?

1. Fetal Alcohol Syndrome is the leading cause of mental retardation in the United States.
2. The risk of an alcoholic woman having a defective child is 35%.
3. Microcephaly, craniofacial malformations, and limb and heart defects are common in affected patients.
4. Short stature and a host of adult maladaptive behaviors have been associated with this syndrome.

129. Which of the following statements is a correct statement about the difference between an Amphetamine-Induced Psychosis and Paranoid Schizophrenia?

1. Paranoid ideation is prominent in the schizophrenic process and not in the Amphetamine-Induced Psychosis.

2. Flattened affect may be prominent in the schizophrenic patient but not in the Amphetamine-Induced Psychosis.
3. Clinically, the Amphetamine-Induced Psychosis can always be differentiated from Paranoid Schizophrenia.
4. Visual hallucinations and hypersexuality may be prominent in the patient with Amphetamine-Induced Psychosis but not in the paranoid schizophrenic patient.

130. Which of the following statements about the epidemiology of cocaine use is/are true?

1. In 1991, 18% of young adults ages 18 to 25 and 26% of adults ages 26 to 34 reported use of cocaine at least once in their lifetimes.
2. Lifetime use of cocaine among adults age 26 and older has steadily increased over the past 20 years.
3. Males are twice as likely as females to have used cocaine in the past month.
4. Use across regions in the United States does not vary at statistically significant levels.

131. Which of the following statements about opioid use is/are true?

1. Demerol (meperidine) is the most commonly used drug among those who use opioids.
2. There are about a half a million opioid users in the United States, scattered around the country.
3. The male-to-female ratio among opioid users is 1:1.
4. The involvement of individuals with opioid dependence in prostitution has played a role in the transmission of HIV.

132. Which of the following statements about the prodromal signs and symptoms of Schizophrenia is/are true?

1. Most often, the prodromal signs are recognized after the diagnosis of Schizophrenia is made.
2. Decreased social and occupational functioning are often noted by friends and family.
3. During the prodromal phase, the individual may develop a new interest in abstract ideas of philosophy.
4. Often schizophrenic individuals have a history of being shy, introverted and passive.

133. Which of the following statements about the use of hospitalization in the treatment of Schizophrenia is/are true?

1. A primary goal of hospitalization may be to establish an effective link between the patient and community services.
2. Hospitalization reduces the stress on the individual and helps with structuring the activities of daily living.
3. Disorganized behavior, suicidal acts or thoughts, and medication stabilization are all reasons to hospitalize the schizophrenic patient.
4. Long-term hospitalization with an emphasis on a custodial approach is more effective than short-term hos-

pitalization with an active, behaviorally oriented approach.

134. Treatment of individuals with a Shared Psychotic Disorder includes which of the following?

1. Separation of the affected person from the dominant partner
2. Psychotherapy of the affected individual, the family, and later the dominant partner
3. Diagnosis and treatment of the psychiatric disorder of the dominant partner
4. Increasing contact with the outside world, which may be useful in preventing a relapse

135. Which of the following statements regarding Delirium is/are true?

1. Disturbances in the sleep–wake cycle are common.
2. Rapid shifts from one emotional state to another may be a feature of Delirium.
3. Usually the electroencephalogram (EEG) is abnormal in delirious patients.
4. The level of alertness in patients is usually unaffected by Delirium.

136. Which of the following statements is/are true?

1. Substance Abuse Disorders are grouped with Delirium, Dementia, and other Cognitive Disorders in DSM-IV.
2. The term "organic mental disorder" is not used in DSM-IV because it implies that only diagnoses in that category have a biological basis.
3. DSM-IV limits the diagnosis of Dementia to "vascular and other causes."
4. Dementia and Amnestic Disorders are in the same group in DSM-IV.

137. Which of the following statements concerning the DSM-IV criteria for Substance Dependence is/are true?

1. The essential feature is a cluster of cognitive, behavioral, and physiological symptoms indicating that the individual continues to use substances despite significant substance-related problems.
2. A diagnosis of Substance Dependence applies to all classes of substances except caffeine.
3. Tolerance indicates a need for greater amounts of a substance to achieve intoxication.
4. Neither withdrawal nor tolerance is sufficient for a diagnosis of Substance Dependence.

138. The diagnosis of Substance Dependence in DSM-IV has six specifiers. Which of the following statements concerning these specifiers is/are true?

1. The four remission specifiers can be applied only after none of the criteria for Substance Dependence or Substance Abuse have been met for at least three months.
2. The first 12 months following Dependence are desig-

nated Early Remission, if no substance use occurs.

3. Early Partial Remission refers to the first six months following cessation of substance use.

4. Sustained Full Remission takes into account the length of time since last use, the total duration of use, and the need for continued evaluation.

139. Regarding DSM-IV diagnosis of Schizophrenia, which of the following statements is/are true?

1. No single symptom is pathognomnic for Schizophrenia.

2. Positive symptoms of Schizophrenia reflect distortion of normal function and negative symptoms reflect the diminution of normal function.

3. Referential delusions are beliefs that general environmental cues are directed specifically at the patient.

4. The characteristic signs and symptoms of Schizophrenia must be present for a significant portion of a one-month period, and some evidence of the disorder must persist for six months.

140. Which of the following negative symptoms of Schizophrenia does the DSM-IV include in its definition of Schizophrenia?

1. Affective flattening
2. Alogia
3. Avolition
4. Anhedonia

141. According to DSM-IV, which of the following characteristics are true of Schizophrenia?

1. Educational progress for individuals with Schizophrenia is frequently disrupted.

2. The majority of individuals with Schizophrenia do marry.

3. The pervasive pattern of problems secondary to Schizophrenia must persist for six months to make the diagnosis.

4. Negative symptoms are uncommon in both the prodromal and residual phases of Schizophrenia.

142. Which of the following statements accurately reflects the description of the course of Schizophrenia in DSM-IV?

1. Schizophrenia is a relentlessly chronic illness.

2. Positive symptoms may become more prominent over the course of the illness.

3. Acute onset predicts a poor prognosis.

4. The median age at onset for the first psychotic episode of Schizophrenia is in the early to mid-20s for men and late 20s for women.

143. DSM-IV lists which of the following characteristics for the diagnosis of the Disorganized Type of Schizophrenia?

1. Disorganized speech
2. Disorganized behavior
3. Flat or inappropriate affect
4. Continuous course without significant remissions

144. The essential features of Schizophreniform Disorder and Schizophrenia in the DSM-IV are:

1. The diagnosis of Schizophreniform Disorder specifically excludes psychotic symptomatology.

2. The total duration of illness for Schizophreniform Disorder is at least one month but less than six months.

3. Schizophreniform Disorder does not include psychotic features.

4. Impairment of social or occupational functioning is not required for a diagnosis of Schizophreniform Disorder.

145. The DSM-IV criteria for the diagnosis of Schizoaffective Disorder include:

1. An uninterrupted period of illness during which, at some time, there is a Major Depressive, Manic, or Mixed Episode concurrent with symptoms that meet Criterion A for Schizophrenia.

2. Delusions and hallucinations occur for at least two weeks during the period of illness in the absence of prominent mood symptoms.

3. Mood symptoms are present for a substantial portion of the entire duration of the illness.

4. Any mood symptoms occurring during a period when Criterion A for Schizophrenia is met qualifies a patient for a diagnosis of Schizoaffective Disorder.

146. The Brief Psychotic Disorder (DSM-IV):

1. Lasts at least one day but not longer than 3 months.

2. May be characterized by rapid shifts from one intense affect to another.

3. Results in residual symptoms once the initial psychotic symptoms abate.

4. May result in a high risk for suicide, especially in younger patients.

147. Psychotic Disorder Due to a General Medical Condition:

1. Is a psychologically mediated psychotic response to be diagnosed with a medical condition.

2. Cannot be due to a brain lesion or insult.

3. Is not associated with hallucinations or delusions.

4. Is the direct physiological result of a medical illness on brain function.

148. Which of the following statements is/are true of a Mixed Episode Mood Disorder?

1. This disorder is characterized by a period in which the criteria for Manic Episode and a Major Depressive Episode are simultaneously met.

2. Some evidence suggests that some individuals may develop a Mixed-like Episode following somatic treatment.

3. Mixed Episodes appear more common in younger individuals.

4. Mixed Episodes may be more common in males than in females.

149. With regards to Major Depressive Disorder, Single Episode or Recurrent:

    1. It has a clinical course of one or more Major Depressive Episodes.
    2. A history of Manic, Mixed, or Hypomanic Episodes precludes a diagnosis of Major Depressive Disorder.
    3. DSM-IV has specifiers for the severity of the current state of the disturbance.
    4. For a particular episode to be considered to have ended, the full criteria for the Major Depressive Episode must not have been met for at least three consecutive months.

150. With regard to Major Depressive Disorder:

    1. It has a typical age onset in the mid-30s.
    2. Some evidence suggests that remissions are shorter early in the illness and longer in the later stages of the illness.
    3. Ten percent of patients with a Major Depressive Episode, Single Episode, are at risk of having a second episode.
    4. About 5–10% of individuals with a Major Depressive Disorder, Single Episode, subsequently develop a Manic Episode and thus have a diagnosis of Bipolar I Disorder.

151. Dysthymic Disorder:

    1. Frequently has a disturbance in sleep architecture as an associated feature.
    2. Develops in equal rates in men and women in adulthood.
    3. Is differentiated from Major Depressive Disorder on the basis of severity.
    4. Is not associated with Axis II disorders.

152. Bipolar I Disorder differs from Bipolar II Disorder in that:

    1. Bipolar I Disorder includes a Manic or Mixed Episode and Bipolar II Disorder does not.
    2. Bipolar II Disorder has Hypomanic Episodes and Bipolar I Disorder does not.
    3. Bipolar I Disorder occurs equally in men and women and Bipolar II Disorder does not.
    4. Psychotic symptoms in the Major Depressive Episode of Bipolar II Disorder are more prominent than in the depressed phase of Bipolar I Disorder.

153. Which of the following statements regarding Bipolar II Disorder is/are true?

    1. The intervals between episodes increases with age.
    2. A minority of individuals with this disorder return to normal function between episodes.
    3. Over the course of five years, half of individuals with this disorder will experience a Manic Episode.
    4. The life time prevalence is 0.5%.

154. Application of the specifier With Melancholic Features is appropriate under which of the following circumstances?

    1. There is a nearly complete absence of pleasure.
    2. Depression is regularly worse in the evening.
    3. There is no affective brightening when circumstances improve or a positive event occurs.
    4. There are clear precipitant(s) for the episode.

155. Longitudinal Course Specifiers for Mood Disorders:

    1. Are applied to the period between the two most recent episodes.
    2. Predict as the best outcome (prognosis) no antecedent Dysthymic Disorder and a period of complete resolution of symptoms between episodes.
    3. Characterize the pattern known as "double depression" as an antecedent Dysthymic Disorder with a Major Depressive Disorder and incomplete resolution of symptoms between episodes.
    4. May be applied to Bipolar I Disorder or Bipolar II Disorder to indicate the presence or absence of symptoms between episodes.

156. Which of the following statements is/are true about the specifier With Rapid Cycling for Mood Disorders?

    1. It applies to situations in which there are six or more episodes meeting the criteria for Major Depressive Episode, Manic Episode, or Mixed Episode in one year.
    2. The symptoms that occur in the episodes in a Rapid Cycling situation are distinctly different from those in a non-Rapid Cycling situation.
    3. Like Bipolar I Disorder, Rapid Cycling is equally divided between males and females.
    4. Rapid Cycling is associated with a poorer prognosis over the long term.

157. Which of the following statements about Agoraphobia is/are true?

    1. In DSM-IV, Agoraphobia is a separate codable diagnosis.
    2. Agoraphobia has as its central feature anxiety about being in places or situations from which escape might be difficult or embarrassing or in which help might not be available should a Panic Attack occur.
    3. Social Phobias and Obsessive-Compulsive Disorders commonly have Agoraphobia as an associated feature.
    4. Patients with Agoraphobia avoid situations where they are alone or endure the situation with much distress.

158. In distinguishing between Panic Disorder With Agoraphobia and Specific Phobia, Situational Type:

    1. With Panic Disorder, the focus of the fear will be on the recurrence of the Panic Attacks rather than on the situation.
    2. The types and number of Panic Attacks with Specific Phobia, Situational Type, will be greater.
    3. Patients with Panic Disorder With Agoraphobia will avoid more situations.

4. The level of intercurrent anxiety will be greater for Specific Phobia, Situational Type.

159. Which of the following statements about Agoraphobia Without History of Panic Disorder is/are true?

1. The disorder is far more common in women.
2. To qualify for this diagnosis, the criteria for Panic Disorder have never been met.
3. The focus of the fear is on the occurrence of incapacitating or extremely embarrassing paniclike symptoms or attacks of limited symptoms rather than a full-blown Panic Attack.
4. In clinical populations, this disorder is more commonly diagnosed than is Panic Disorder With Agoraphobia.

160. Specific Phobias:

1. Are more frequently diagnosed in women.
2. Most frequently have their onset in childhood.
3. For the Situational Type have a bimodal age of onset with one peak in childhood and another in the mid-20s.
4. May have particularly strong familial patterns when of the Blood-Injection-Injury Type.

161. Which of the following statements concerning Obsessive-Compulsive Disorder is/are true?

1. Males have this diagnosis more frequently than do females.
2. By definition, adults with this disorder have at some time in the course of illness recognized the unreasonable nature of their obsessions and compulsions.
3. Individuals with this disorder are drawn toward situations that involve the content of the obsession.
4. Individuals with Tourette's Disorder have a high incidence of Obsessive-Compulsive Disorder.

162. Which of the following statements is/are true of Post-traumatic Stress Disorder (PTSD):

1. Diminished responsiveness to the external world and/or decreased interest or participation in previously enjoyable events is evidenced.
2. The affected individual has persistent symptoms of anxiety or arousal that were not present before the trauma.
3. Affected individuals may experience a foreshortened view of the future.
4. The severity, duration, and proximity of the individual's exposure to the trauma are important factors in developing this disorder.

163. The DSM-IV diagnosis of Acute Stress Disorder differs from that of PTSD in which of the following ways?

1. With Acute Stress Disorder, the symptoms occur within one month of the experience of the traumas, whereas with PTSD the onset of symptoms may be delayed for months or years.

2. The traumatic events that cause Acute Stress Disorder are less severe than those that result in PTSD.
3. Dissociative symptoms are more prominent in Acute Stress Disorder than in PTSD.
4. Individuals with Acute Stress Disorder do not reexperience the traumatic event via intrusive recollection or dreams, whereas individuals with PTSD do.

164. Which of the following statements about Generalized Anxiety Disorder is/are true?

1. Children with this disorder tend to be overly conforming, perfectionistic, and unsure of themselves.
2. In community samples, the lifetime prevalence is about 5%.
3. Studies have failed to identify a clear genetic pattern in families.
4. Women and men are diagnosed with this disorder with equal frequency.

165. Which of the following medical conditions could result in a DSM-IV diagnosis of Anxiety Disorder Due to a General Medical Condition?

1. Thyroid condition
2. Thiamine deficiency
3. Congestive heart failure
4. HIV infection

166. Which of the following statements is/are true of Somatization Disorder?

1. Symptoms of this disorder are not influenced by culture.
2. The course of the illness is characterized by episodes of intense symptomatology with long periods of complete remission of symptoms between episodes.
3. It only rarely occurs in female first-degree relatives of women with this disorder.
4. This diagnosis is rarely made in men in the United States.

167. Which of the following statements is/are true of Undifferentiated Somatoform Disorder?

1. One or more physical complaints persist for six months or more.
2. This is a residual category for persistent somatoform presentations that do not meet the criteria for Somatization Disorder.
3. The most frequent complaints are chronic fatigue, loss of appetite, and gastrointestinal or genitourinary symptoms.
4. Neurasthenia would be classified as this disorder according to DSM-IV.

168. Which of the following statements is/are true of Pain Disorder?

1. Pain Disorders are frequently associated with Depressive Disorders and Anxiety Disorders.
2. DSM-IV defines "acute" in regard to this diagnosis as 1 year or less.

3. Psychological factors are judged to play a significant role in the onset, severity, exacerbation, or maintenance of the pain.
4. Individuals with this disorder cannot have evidence of anatomical or physiological pathology.

169. Which of the following statements regarding the Body Dysmorphic Disorder is/are true?

1. The most common perceived defect by individuals with this disorder involves the face.
2. This disorder may result in extreme social isolation.
3. Individuals with this disorder frequently feel that others are taking special notice of their defect.
4. Individuals with this disorder eagerly discuss the defect with their physician.

170. Which of the following statements regarding Dissociative Disorders is/are true?

1. Dissociation is a disruption of the normally integrated functions of consciousness, memory, and identity.
2. A Dissociative Disorder may have a sudden or gradual onset, and be transient or chronic in course.
3. Dissociative symptoms may be present in other disorders, such as Acute Stress Disorder and Posttraumatic Stress Disorder.
4. Dissociation is inherently pathological and always is indicative of psychopathology.

171. Which of the following statements about Dissociative Amnesia is/are true?

1. This disorder occurs exclusively in adults.
2. This disorder usually occurs spontaneously without environmental stimuli playing a role.
3. Individuals with this disorder are unaware of their memory problems.

4. The essential feature is one or more episodes of the failure to recall important personal information that is too extensive to be explained by ordinary forgetfulness.

172. Which of the following statements is/are true of Sexual Aversion Disorder?

1. The essential feature is aversion to and active avoidance of genital sexual contact.
2. The affected individual may experience revulsion to all aspects of sexuality, including kissing and touching.
3. The aversion may be to specific aspects of sexuality (secretions, penetration).
4. Covert strategies, such as excessive work, going to sleep early, and neglecting one's personal appearance, may be employed to avoid sexual activity.

173. Which of the following statements about Sexual Arousal Disorders is/are true?

1. In males and females, this diagnosis refers to an inability to become sexually aroused at a psychological level.
2. Both men and women who have this disorder have some physiological inability that interferes with intercourse.
3. Men with this disorder are always impotent.
4. Anxiety, fear of failure, and concern about sexual performance play significant roles in this disorder.

174. Which of the following statements is/are true about the DSM-IV diagnosis of Dyspareunia?

1. This disorder occurs only in women.
2. Vaginismus and lack of lubrication are common causes.
3. The pain is experienced only during intercourse.
4. In women, the pain may be described as superficial at intromission and deep during thrusting.

# ANSWERS AND EXPLANATIONS

1. Answer is **d**. Although disorientation to time, place, and situation is common, few patients will be disoriented to person. The old and the young are especially susceptible to delirium, with the elderly being the most vulnerable. At least 10% of the hospitalized elderly have delirium. Some patients have hallucinations as a feature of delirium. (*DSM-IV 124–126*)

2. Answer is **c**. The psychotic symptoms present in delirium are fragmented, and unsystematized and occur in the clinical context of impaired cognitive ability. Laboratory studies of electrolytes, drug screens, etc., are important data in the assessment of the delirious patient. Preexisting dementia or other intracranial pathology will increase a patient's vulnerability to delirium. Delirious patients always have difficulty in focusing or shifting their attention. In the emergency room setting, Malingering and Factitious Disorder must be ruled out and the unusual presentation and lack of laboratory abnormalities will make this differential diagnosis an easy task. (*DSM-IV 124–126*)

3. Answer is **b**. Demented patients are alert and do not have the fluctuating level of consciousness associated with delirium. Multiple cognitive impairments, including memory impairment, aphasia, agnosia, apraxia, or a disturbance in executive function, are the essential features of dementia. All of these impairments represent a decline from previous levels of functioning. (*DSM-IV 133–135*)

4. Answer is **a**. Apraxia, aphasia, and disorders of executive function are characteristic of dementia and not of Amnestic Disorders as described in DSM-IV. Patients with Amnestic Disorders have an impaired ability to learn new information or to recall previously learned material. Affected individuals have a severe memory disturbance that may result in disorientation to place and time, but rarely to person. Patients will deny their problems, and this may cause problems with their environment. (*DSM-IV 156–158*)

5. Answer is **e**. A documented medical disorder that has a direct physiological link to the psychiatric symptom is needed to make the diagnosis of a Mental Disorder Due to a General Medical Condition. The clinician must be alert to symptoms that are atypical for primary mental disorders, such as unusual age of onset. (*DSM-IV 165-169*)

6. Answer is **a**. Cognitive decline is not a feature of the diagnosis Personality Change Due to a General Medical Disorder. The patient with this diagnosis exhibits uncharacteristic behavior that is a deviation from a stable personality structure. Emotional lability, poor impulse con-

trol, and outbursts of rage or aggression may be present. As the name of the disorder indicates, this personality change is the direct result of a physiological change due to a medical disorder. The essence of this diagnosis is that it is a departure from a previously stable personality pattern. (*DSM-IV 171–174*)

7. Answer is **d**. The diagnoses of Substance Abuse and Substance Dependence are mutually exclusive. Criterion B states that symptoms listed in Criteria A have never met the criteria for Substance Dependence. The diagnosis of Substance Abuse does not apply to nicotine or caffeine and does not include tolerance or withdrawal. The episodes of role failure, being in physically hazardous situations, and/or having legal problems recurrent over a 12-month period are related to substance abuse. (*DSM-IV 182–183*)

8. Answer is **b**. Persons with Schizophrenia can have a variety of perceptual disturbances, with auditory hallucinations by far the most common. They experience these voices as separate and distinct from their own thoughts. Negative or threatening voices are quite common, and the experience of having a voice(s) offering a running commentary on the patient's behavior is considered to be so characteristic of Schizophrenia that it fully satisfies criteria A. Not all hallucinations are indicative of pathology. In some cultures, hallucinatory experiences are part of religious ceremony. The common experiences of hypnogogic (going to sleep) or hypnopompic (waking up) hallucinations are within the realm of normal experience. (*DSM-IV 273–278*)

9. Answer is **e**. The speech patterns of all patients reflect patterns of thought, and the communication problems of patients with Schizophrenia clearly demonstrate this situation. A disorganized, idiosyncratic mode of communication can be readily observed in many such patients. DSM-IV makes a distinction between grossly disorganized behavior and simply aimless or seemingly purposeless behavior. The rationale seems to be that the behavioral diagnostic criteria should not be too broadly interpreted. Catatonic behavior occurs in a wide range of conditions and not exclusively in Schizophrenia. Goal-directed behavior may be especially problematic for persons with Schizophrenia. (*DSM-IV 276–277*)

10. Answer is **a**. Lack of insight may be the best predictor of poor outcome, perhaps owing to its role in noncompliance. Difficulty concentrating is a common problem, and may be due to the distraction of internal stimuli. Affective symptoms may the best predictor of suicidal potential.

Day–night reversal is not uncommon. Somatic delusions are not included in the list of outcome predictors. (*DSM-IV 283*)

11. Answer is **b**. Young men under the age of 30 with depressive symptoms, and recently discharged from the hospital with no employment prospects seem to have the greatest risk for suicide. Approximately 10% of persons with Schizophrenia kill themselves. (*DSM-IV 280*)

12. Answer is **c**. DSM-IV increased the length of time for active symptoms from the one week of DSM-III-R to four weeks (one month). This should reduce the number of false positive diagnoses of Schizophrenia. (*DSM-IV 285*)

13. Answer is **d**. The first-degree biological relatives of an individual with Schizophrenia have a risk for Schizophrenia that is 10 times greater than that of the general population. Typically, Schizophrenia is a disorder of late adolescence and younger adulthood, although exceptions exist. Significant differences exist between male and female patients with Schizophrenia, although a difference in the sex ratio of those affected is difficult to document. Women tend to have a later onset, more affective symptoms, and a better outcome. Many factors influence the diagnosis of Schizophrenia, however, when these differences are taken into account, the lifetime prevalence is estimated to be 0.5%–1%. (*DSM-IV 282–283*)

14. Answer is **b**. Negative symptoms and disorganized thinking are less likely in late-onset Schizophrenia and paranoid delusions and hallucinations are more common. More women are represented in the population of late-onset Schizophrenia, and their occupational history tends to be better. The course of late-onset Schizophrenia tends to be chronic, however, a good response to neuroleptics at lower doses is frequently seen. (*DSM-IV 281*)

15. Answer is **d**. The distinguishing characteristics of the Paranoid Type of Schizophrenia tend to be stable over time. Individuals with this disorder tend to have a later age at onset and a better prognosis. Prominent delusions and hallucinations play central roles in the disorder. The delusions frequently have a coherent core and are most often of a persecutory or grandiose type. These individuals may be angry, aloof, haughty, or argumentative. Also, a stilted formal tone may pervade their interactions with others. (*DSM-IV 287–288*)

16. Answer is **a**. Catalepsy, not cataplexy, is characteristic of this diagnosis. The former term refers to the "waxy flexibility" that many of these patients demonstrate, and the latter term refers to the extreme weakness of antigravity muscles seen with narcolepsy, for example. Catatonic excitement is excessive motoric activity seemingly unrelated to external stimuli. Extreme negativism and posturing are also characteristic of this disorder. The mean-ingless repetition of a word or phrase spoken by another person is echolalia, and the imitations of the movements of others is echopraxia. Both are characteristic of the disorder. (*DSM-IV 288–289*)

17. Answer is **b**. Mood disturbances do not play a major role in this disorder, and according to the criteria, they must not. Typically, one or more nonbizarre delusions are present and well circumscribed. Behavior is not odd or bizarre, and symptoms of Schizophrenia, such as prominent auditory or visual hallucinations, are absent. If a patient has ever met Criterion A for Schizophrenia, the diagnosis of Delusional Disorder cannot be made. Tactile and olfactory hallucinations may be present and prominent, especially if related to delusional material. (*DSM-IV 296–297*)

18. Answer is **a**. The types of Delusional Disorder are: Erotomanic, Grandiose, Jealous, Persecutory, Somatic, Mixed, and Unspecified. Erotomanic types have delusions that another person is in love with them, whereas a jealous type has delusions that a sexual partner is unfaithful. Grandiose types have delusions of inflated worth, power, etc., or of a special relationship with a deity or powerful person. Persecutory types have delusions of a malevolent conspiracy against them; somatic types have delusions that a physical defect or general medical condition afflicts them. Mixed types have delusions with characteristics of more than one type, without a dominant theme. (*DSM-IV 297–298*)

19. Answer is **d**. Usually this disorder begins when one of the pair (the primary case) has a delusional system that he or she imposes on a passive partner. When the two persons are separated, the passive partner's delusional system will diminish or disappear. The shared delusion(s) can be of any type, and are not limited to a particular theme. The primary case can have any psychotic disorder, including Schizophrenia. (*DSM-IV 305–306*)

20. Answer is **e**. According to DSM-IV, depressive symptoms must be present for two weeks, not four weeks. Sleep disturbances, fatigue, and loss of energy are frequently reported in depressed individuals, and sleep EEGs clearly document sleep abnormalities. Interest in previously pleasurable activities, including sexuality, are markedly diminished. A decreased ability to attend and to concentrate also frequently accompanies a Major Depressive Episode. (*DSM-IV 320–323*)

21. Answer is **a**. DSM-IV determines that a week of manic symptoms is necessary to meet the criteria. If the symptoms are of such a severity as to warrant hospitalization, then less time is required to meet the time threshold. Some 50% to 60% of patients with a Manic Episode will experience a Major Depressive Episode immediately preceding or following the Manic Episode. Frequently, the

symptoms apparent during a Manic Episode reach a psychotic level. Grandiose delusions would be a common example. During Manic Episodes, patients frequently deny that they are behaving uncharacteristically or are in need of care. Attempts to intervene will often result in angry, occasionally violent, outbursts from the patient. Depressive and manic symptoms may frequently coexist in patients. (*DSM-IV 328–329*)

22. Answer is **d**. DSM-IV specifically excludes delusions and hallucinations from its diagnosis of Hypomanic Episode. The Hypomanic Episode is a distinct period during which there is a mood disturbance characterized by a persistent irritability or alternating euphoria and irritability that lasts for at least four days. The mood and associated behavioral changes are a departure from normal functioning and are readily apparent to others. The development of a Hypomanic Episode is not always associated with social or occupational impairment, and affected individuals may be unusually productive. However, the Hypomanic Episode is clearly distinct from the individual's normal mood and is readily observed by others who know the person well. (*DSM-IV 335*)

23. Answer is **b**. The prevalence rates for Major Depressive Disorder appear to be unrelated to ethnicity, education, income, or marital status. The lifetime risk for this disorder in community samples is 10–25% for women and 5–12% for men. Major Depressive Disorder is associated with high mortality, with 15% of severely affected patients dying by suicide. Postpubertal females have twice the rate of the disorder as men. In prepubertal children, no gender difference is noted. Chronic medical conditions commonly are associated with Major Depressive Disorder. Examples include diabetes, stroke, myocardial infarction, and AIDS. (*DSM-IV 340*)

24. Answer is **a**. The severity of an initial episode does predict for the persistence of symptoms. Naturalistic follow-up studies suggest that 40% of patients one year after diagnosis still meet the criteria for Major Depressive Episode. Partial remission following an episode increases the likelihood of both additional episodes and a persistence of symptoms between episodes. Thus, the course specifiers of "With Full Interepisode Recovery" and "Without Full Interepisode Recovery" may have predictive value. Severe psychosocial stressors, such as the loss of a loved one or divorce, may precede the onset of a Major Depressive Disorder, but play a lesser role later in the course of the disorder. Mood Disorders tend to follow familial patterns, and first-degree relatives have a 1.5 to three times greater risk than does the general population for developing a Major Depressive Disorder. (*DSM-IV 342*)

25. Answer is **c**. Persons with Dysthymic Disorder experience chronic depression as a usual part of their personal being. The depressive features are incorporated into the patient's identity. Feelings of inadequacy, low energy, loss of interest in pleasure, social withdrawal, and guilt may dominate the clinical picture in the patient with Dysthymic Disorder. Vegetative symptoms seem to be less common. For DSM-IV diagnosis, the patient must experience depressive symptoms most of the day on most days for two years, as well as associated symptoms, such as sleep disturbance, poor self-esteem, or appetite disturbance. The lifetime prevalence for this disorder is 6%, the point prevalence is 3%. (*DSM-IV 345–346*)

26. Answer is **c**. The first episode of this disorder is more likely to be a manic episode if the patient is a male. The vast majority of patients who have a Manic Episode go on to have one or more episodes in the future. Most Manic Episodes precede a Major Depressive Episode. Women with the disorder may have a greater risk of developing subsequent episodes in the postpartum period. By definition, rapid cycling refers to the having of four or more episodes in a given year. (*DSM-IV 353*)

27. Answer is **d**. Late adolescence or early adulthood is the typical age of onset for this disorder. Its onset may be early enough in life that the cyclothymic symptoms are mistaken for inherent temperament. For this diagnosis to apply, the individual must have only cyclothymic symptoms for at least two years and not have Major Depressive Manic or Mixed Episode. After two years of symptoms, the development of a Major Depressive Episode would result in the patient's diagnosis being Cyclothymic Disorder and Bipolar II Disorder. (*DSM-IV 363*)

28. Answer is **a**. Individuals with Atypical Features have an extreme sensitivity to rejection from others and to external circumstances. Unlike the patients with Melancholic Features, these patients will have significant affective and mood brightening to positive events that lasts for extended periods if the situation remains positive. This sensitivity to rejection has an early onset, and individuals may avoid relationships because of it. Hypersomnia, increased appetite and weight gain, and leaden paralysis are all common Atypical Features. These features occur more commonly in women and younger individuals and may have an earlier age of onset, with a more chronic and less episodic course. (*DSM-IV 384–385*)

29. Answer is **b**. Younger individuals appear to be at higher risk for winter depressive episodes. If the Seasonal Episode is more linked to psychosocial stressors, such as seasonal unemployment, this specifier should not be used. Women make up 60–90% of cases, but whether this represents the well-known increased risk that women have for Major Depressive Disorder or an additional risk for women is not clear. The clinician should evaluate the preceding two years for evidence of seasonal mood variations before applying this specifier. Increased appetite

associated with weight gain and a craving for carbohydrates, hypersomnia, and low energy are frequent characteristics of the Major Depressive Episodes associated with this specifier. (*DSM-IV 389*)

30. Answer is **e**. The differential diagnosis of Panic Attack is complicated by several factors. First, no exclusive relationship exists between the type of Panic Attack and specific Anxiety or other disorders. Second, some Anxiety Disorders require the presence of specific types of Panic Attacks, but patients may report experiencing both required types and other types. For example, Panic Disorder requires the experience of unexpected Panic Attacks, but patients with Panic Disorder frequently report having situation-bound attacks. Many patients experience limited symptom attacks, but do not experience four of the required 13 cognitive/somatic symptoms. Patients with Social or Specific Phobias may experience situation-bound Panic Attacks. These patients often can readily identify the trigger that initiated the Panic Attack and will avoid such situations. (*DSM-IV 394–395*)

31. Answer is **e**. The age of onset of Panic Disorder is primarily in late adolescence, with a smaller peak in the mid-30's. DSM-IV criteria are unexpected Panic Attacks followed by at least one month of concern about having more attacks or about the consequence of having attacks, or behavioral alterations due to the attacks. Aside from anxiety related to their Panic Attacks, many patients report increased anxiety unrelated to any particular stimulus. Worries about the outcome of routine events and catastrophizing ordinary occurrences are common in patients with Panic Disorder. Major Depressive Disorder occurs frequently in patients with Panic Disorder. Some 50% to 60% of patients will have both disorders at some point in the course of the illness. One third of patients with Panic Disorder will have a Major Depressive Disorder preceding the development of Panic Disorder. (*DSM-IV 397–398*)

32. Answer is **a**. Having a Specific Phobia of one type increases the likelihood of having another Specific Phobia of the same type (e.g., cats and snakes). If the fear, however intense, is experienced only in the presence of the specific stimulus and that stimulus is not present, the fear of the stimulus causes no restrictions, and the patient is not distressed by the fear, then the criteria for social and/or occupational dysfunction are not met and thus a Specific Phobia is not diagnosed. Typically, adolescents and adults with this disorder recognize that the fear is excessive and unreasonable; however, children do not. In adult clinical settings, the correct sequence of most to least frequent type is Situational, Natural Environment, Blood-Injection-Injury, and Animal. Animal and Natural Environment Specific Phobias frequently begin in childhood. (*DSM-IV 405-406*)

33. Answer is **b**. Persons with this diagnosis often have much anticipatory anxiety about upcoming social or performance events. They may experience a great deal of anxiety far in advance of these events. The essential feature is the fear of social or performance situations that would lead to embarrassment. The disorder has roots in childhood, with affected adults reporting timidity and shyness as childhood characteristics. Affected adults may have poor social skills, few friends, and unfulfilling relationships. Low self-esteem and underachievement are also common associated features. Although epidemiological studies show that more women than men have the disorder, clinical studies indicate an equal distribution among men and women or a preponderance of men. (*DSM-IV 411–412*)

34. Answer is **d**. Individuals with this disorder experience mounting tension or anxiety that is relieved by yielding to the compulsion, and thus the anxiety is experienced before the compulsive act. The modal age of onset for males is 6 to 16 years and for females it is 20 to 29 years. Typically, the disorder begins insidiously and follows a waxing and waning course. Over time, the individual may incorporate the obsessions and compulsions his or her into daily routine. Common themes in obsessions are contamination, doubts, a need for a particular order of things, and aggressive or hostile urges. Evidence is accumulating that supports a biological underpinning for this disorder. A higher concordance rate for monozygotic twins than for dizygotic twins is an example of such evidence. (*DSM-IV 420*)

35. Answer is **a**. DSM-IV criteria for this disorder include such events as the diagnosis of a life-threatening event. Persons with the disorder typically avoid all stimuli associated with the event, making deliberate efforts to avoid thoughts, feelings, or conversations about it. The traumatic event produced intense fear, helplessness, and/or horror in the affected individuals that typically is reexperienced. Although some will develop symptoms quickly after the event, a significant number will have a delayed onset of six months or more after the trauma. (*DSM-IV 424–425*)

36. Answer is **c**. During the course of the disorder, the focus may shift from one concern to another. Most individuals with this disorder do not experience their worry or anxiety as excessive and feel that their anxiety is appropriate. Many other associated symptoms frequently accompany the disorder. Comorbidity with Mood Disorders is very common, especially with Depressive Disorders. Patients also complain of poor sleep, chronic fatigue, and muscle tension regularly. DSM-IV states that the essential feature of the disorder is excessive worry or anxiety occurring over more days than not over a six-month period. (*DSM-IV 432–433*)

37. Answer is **c**. Many types of anxiety may be manifest with this disorder, but phobic behavior does not dominate the picture. When making this diagnosis, the clinician must make two judgments: whether the symptoms of anxiety are in excess of what could be expected from a withdrawal or intoxication syndrome, and whether the anxiety symptoms are of such a degree as to merit specific clinical attention. Many substances, such as caffeine, marijuana, cocaine, volatile inhalants, and heavy metals may cause the clinical picture. This disorder does not occur exclusively within the course of a delirium, according to DSM-IV. (*DSM-IV 441*)

38. Answer is **a**. Actually, the somatic complaints must begin before age 30. The essential feature of this disorder is a pattern of recurring multiple, clinically significant, and somatic complaints in the absence of demonstrable clinical disease. The somatic complaints are usually vague, ill defined and involve many organ systems. DSM-IV divides the complaints into four symptom groups: pain, gastrointestinal, sexual, and pseudoneurological. It specifies the number of symptoms, usually excluding pain, under each of these headings. (*DSM-IV 449–450*)

39. Answer is **d**. Typically, a conversion "seizure" varies from one episode to the next and lacks the stereotypic presentation of physiologically based seizure activity. Quite frequently, conversion symptoms involve voluntary muscle or sensory modalities. Various types of "paralysis" and "anesthesia" may result that do not follow anatomical patterns or physiological mechanisms. Caution must be exercised when making this diagnosis. One third of individuals with conversion symptoms may have a current or prior neurological condition. Certain neurological disorders, such as multiple sclerosis, may appear to be a Conversion Disorder, and thus a careful and thorough evaluation of the patient must be done. DSM-IV acknowledges the role of psychological factors in the genesis of the disorder, requiring that psychological factors be associated with the onset or exacerbation of conversion symptoms. (DSM-IV 452–453)

40. Answer is **b**. Conversion Disorders in children under the age of 10 are usually limited to gait problems and seizures. The age of onset is usually from age 10 to age 35, although new-onset conversion may occur late in life. Individuals in rural areas, of lower socioeconomic status, and in developing regions have higher rates of this disorder. The form of conversion symptoms is frequently dictated by cultural norms about the expression of distress. In some cases, culture-bound conversion symptoms are observed. Women are more frequently diagnosed with the disorder than men and they experience more symptoms on the left side of the body than on the right. Men with this diagnosis have a higher rate of Antisocial Disorder as an associated disorder. In men, this diagnosis must be differentiated from Malingering. (*DSM-IV 454–455*)

41. Answer is **b**. The concern and preoccupation are not of delusional intensity. The affected individual retains the ability to acknowledge that he or she may be exaggerating the extent of the feared disease or that there is no disease at all. However, persons with this diagnosis are very preoccupied with their physical well-being and the possibility of undetected disease. Repeated physical and laboratory examinations that reveal no pathology do little to allay the concerns of the patient. Strained doctor–patient relations often result, and patients may doctor-shop in their quest for validation of their fears. Serious childhood illness and illness in family members may set the stage for the development of this disorder. This diagnosis occurs equally in males and females and has a typical age of onset in early adulthood. These patients are usually quite resistant to mental health referral. (*DSM-IV 463–465*)

42. Answer is **e**. For these individuals, the assuming of the patient role is the central motivation for their behavior. Freedom from responsibility, economic gain, or other external incentives are not a part of this clinical picture. Patients with the disorder may have a dramatic, although quite vague and contradictory, presentation. Frequent complaints of pain and the subsequent administration of narcotic analgesics may pose problems in the longer-term management of these patients. Extensive medical treatment in childhood or during adolescence may predispose individuals for the development of this condition. The phenomenon of approximate answers (1 + 1 = 3, or "The color of snow is blue") may be a feature associated with this condition. (*DSM-IV 471–473*)

43. Answer is **a**. Localized amnesia results in a failure to recall events that occurred during a specific period of time, usually the first few hours following a profoundly disturbing event. Selective amnesia closely resembles the localized type, except that the affected individual remembers some but not all of the events occurring in a circumscribed span of time. Generalized and systematized amnesias are less common, but result in the loss of all recall of one's entire life with the generalized type and of categories of information with the systematized type. (*DSM-IV 478*)

44. Answer is **b**. Although the assumption of a new identity is not common during fugue states, when it is assumed, the new identity is usually more gregarious and uninhibited than the prefugue personality. Dissociative Fugue has sudden, expected travel as an essential feature, sometimes resulting in months of long-distance traveling covering thousands of miles. During the fugue state, the individual appears to be free of psychopathology, may engage in complex social activities, and attracts no untoward attention. Upon return to the prefugue state, the entire content of the fugue state is lost and no memory of it is retained. Recovering from fugue states usually is rapid, although unusual cases may persist. (*DSM-IV 481–483*)

45. Answer is **c**. The primary identity that carries the individual's given name is usually depressed, dependent, guilty, and passive. The alternative identities are most often in stark contrast to this primary identity. More passive alternative identities tend to have a less well-defined personal history and memory. More aggressive or hostile alternative personalities tend to have more complete memories and identities. Transition from one personality to another is often triggered by psychosocial stress, and usually there are 10 or fewer alternative personalities. The essential feature of this disorder is the failure of integration of memory, identity, and consciousness. (*DSM-IV 484– 485*)

46. Answer is **c**. During depersonalization episodes, the individual retains intact reality testing and is able to discern that the feelings of detachment and estrangement from self are only feelings and do not represent reality. Depersonalization episodes are quite common both in individuals with mental disorders and in the general population. As many as half of the adult population may have experienced a depersonalization episode in severe stress. Standardized testing reveals that persons with the disorder are highly hypnotizable and have high dissociative capacity. (*DSM-1V 488– 489*)

47. Answer is **b**. While in some individuals the low sexual desire may be global, it may be limited to a particular partner or situation. In general, an absence or deficiency of sexual fantasies or desire characterizes this disorder. These individuals do not seek or initiate sexual contact, and thus tension may develop in a couple. The clinician should carefully assess both partners to gauge their sexual expectations in the context of the couple relationship. Usually this disorder develops in adulthood in response to stress or interpersonal difficulties. (*DSM-IV 496– 497*)

48. Answer is **a**. Males with Male Orgasmic Disorder most commonly do not achieve orgasm during intercourse, but can do so with manual or oral stimulation. Female Orgasmic Disorder is more prevalent in younger women and tends to have been lifelong. Orgasmic capacity increases with age in females, and once orgasm has been attained, it is uncommon to lose that capacity. With males, increasing age may decrease orgasmic capacity, and so age should be taken into account when evaluating a male. (*DSM-IV 505–509*)

49. Answer is **b**. The majority of males with this disorder can delay orgasm when self-masturbating. A number of factors enter into the clinical evaluation of the disorder, including age, novelty of the situation, frequency of sexual activity, and amount of sexual experience. The attainment of orgasm before penetration or before the patient wishes it is the cardinal symptom of the disorder. The partners' evaluation of the lapse of time between the initiation of sexual activity and the attainment of orgasm is important. Inexperienced young males are most typically affected. (*DSM-IV 509–510*)

50. Answer is **c**. A true Manic Episode is associated with inflated self-esteem and grandiosity. Other symptoms include decreased need for sleep, pressure of speech, flight of ideas, distractibility, psychomotor agitation, and sexual acting out. Such symptoms may also be the direct effects of antidepressant medication or steroids. (*SP 328– 329*)

51. Answer is **a**. The term "anorexia" is a misnomer, since these individuals do experience hunger. The cardinal feature of the disorder is the refusal to maintain a body weight that is about 85% of the weight considered to be normal for an individual of a certain age and height. These individuals are intensely fearful of gaining weight and will take extreme measures to prevent weight gain. Occasionally, these weight-reduction measures will result in death. A disturbance in the perception of body shape or size is another central feature. For example, the affected person will point to an emaciated limb and complain about how fat it is. Significant neuroendocrine abnormalities result from starvation, and individuals with this disorder are no exception. The cessation of menses is a well-known effect of starvation. (*DSM-IV 539–540*)

52. Answer is **c**. Individuals with Anorexia Nervosa may be obsessed with food and food-related activities. Cooking, recipe collecting, and food hoarding may all be associated with the diagnosis. Usually the family is the source of the impetus for the individual to seek treatment. Only rarely will the affected person complain of the weight loss. Different methods are used to decrease food intake. Some persons will become ever more restrictive of the amount and the type of food they consume. Others may alternately binge and purge. Diuretics and laxatives may be abused. This disorder is far more common in industrialized societies and in females. The mean age of onset is 17, and only rarely is the diagnosis made before puberty or after the age of 40. (*DSM-IV 540–543*)

53. Answer is **b**. Persons with this disorder may be underweight, overweight, or of normal weight. The disorder is most common in industrialized countries and has a prevalence of about 1–3% in female adolescents and young adult women. Depressive and anxious symptoms frequently accompany the diagnosis. A central feature of the disorder is the excessive emphasis on body shape and size in self-evaluation. (*DSM-IV 545–546*)

54. Answer is **c**. Most REM sleep is in the last third of sleep, and most slow-wave sleep is in the first one third of sleep. REM follows a cyclic pattern that is predictable and occurs at 80–100-minute intervals. Sleep architecture is complex, but can be divided into REM sleep and stages 1–4. Understanding the structure of sleep is essential when diagnosing and treating sleep disorders. More time is spent in stage 2 sleep (about 50%) than in any other sleep stage. Children and adolescents have stable sleep

patterns, with regular and predictable deep sleep stages. With increasing age, there is a deterioration of sleep continuity and depth. (*DSM-IV 551–552*)

55. Answer is **d**. Sleep studies of elderly women show better preservation of sleep continuity and slow-wave sleep than in elderly men. The discrepancy between the data and complaints has yet to be explained. The onset is usually sudden, often at a time of stress, such as a medical illness with an initial phase of progressively worsening symptoms followed by a chronic period of sleep problems that linger long after the stress has resolved. In clinics that specialize in the treatment of sleep disorders, 15–25% of the patients will have a diagnosis of Primary Insomnia. (*DSM-IV 553–555*)

56. Answer is **c**. The daytime naps of individuals with a diagnosis of Primary Hypersomnia are slow and gradual in onset. The naps are of long duration and lack a refreshing quality. Following nocturnal sleep or a nap, the individual is slow to arouse and remains sleepy for a significant length of time after the sleep event. The initial sleep event is 8–12 hours and has a normal architecture. Approximately 5–10% of patients in sleep disorder clinics carry this diagnosis. (*DSM-IV 557–558*)

57. Answer is **d**. Persons with untreated Narcolepsy average two to six sleep attacks a day. These sleep attacks are irresistible, usually last 10 to 20 minutes and are experienced by the individual as refreshing. Cataplexy and sleep paralysis are disturbing, although benign, associated symptoms of Narcolepsy. Intense emotion will tend to bring on a cataplectic attack. Sleep paralysis is especially disturbing to the patient since the patient is fully awake but unable to move. Also disturbing are the sleep-emergence (hypnopompic) hallucinations or the sleep-onset (hypnagogic) hallucinations. These phenomena may represent the intrusion of REM sleep elements into the waking state. (*DSM-IV 562–564*)

58. Answer is **e**. These individuals may be very restless during the apnea episodes, with violent, flailing body movements. They have frequent partial arousals during the night owing to problems with their breathing. Daytime sleepiness due to these sleep interruptions is the usual presenting complaint. Daytime naps will be unrefreshing, and will often be followed by a dull headache upon awakening. Since many of these individuals breathe through their mouths during sleep, severe drying of the oral mucosa can result, and the person may get up to drink liquids during the night to relieve the dryness. (*DSM-IV 567–570*)

59. Answer is **d**. The essential feature of this disorder is the mismatch of the individual's circadian rhythm and the demands of the environment. Rotating shifts are notorious for causing this problem. When given the opportunity,

these individuals will go to bed later and arise later, typically on weekends or on vacation. The Jet Lag and Shift Work types are more common in the "morning person." The person with the Delayed Sleep Phase Type may have characteristics associated with the schizoid, schizotypal, or avoidant personality. (*DSM-IV 573–576*)

60. Answer is **b**. The individual with this disorder will be fully awake upon emerging from a nightmare. The essential element of the diagnosis is the repeated occurrence of frightening dream sequences that awaken the person from sleep. Typically, the person remembers the dream in detail and has these dreams in the last half of sleep, since that is when most REM sleep occurs. Nightmares occur only during REM sleep. (*DSM-IV 580*)

61. Answer is **d**. In contrast to the Nightmare Disorder, Sleep Terror Disorder occurs during non-REM sleep, usually during stage 3 or 4. The person usually abruptly cries out, is difficult to comfort or arouse, and usually goes back to sleep readily after the episode. The next morning the person will generally have little or no recollection of the previous night's events. Typically, the disorder begins in childhood and resolves spontaneously in adolescence. In adults, the disorder may begin between the ages of 20 and 30 and will follow a chronic course. (*DSM-IV 583–585*)

62. Answer is **b**. The individual with this diagnosis may exhibit impulsivity or aggressiveness between episodes. Data on the prevalence of the diagnosis are limited, but it apparently is rare. The essential feature is the failure to resist aggressive impulses that occur in discrete episodes. These episodes are typically preceded by a sense of rising tension or arousal that is relieved immediately following the episode. Later, the individual may experience a sense of remorse or embarrassment. The aggression expressed during an episode is grossly out of proportion to any stimulus that preceded the episode. (*DSM-IV 609–611*)

63. Answer is **d**. DSM-IV specifically excludes individuals who are responding to psychotic perceptual disturbance, as well as those who set fires for monetary gain, for political motives, or for the concealment of criminal activity. In spite of the fact that 40% of all cases of Pyromania involved persons under the age of 18, it is still a rare disorder in children. Individuals may make extensive plans before setting a fire, and may be in the audience watching the fire. These individuals are often preoccupied with fire and fire-related activities. They may spend time at the local firehouse, collect paraphernalia related to fire, and even become firefighters. (*DSM-IV 614–615*)

64. Answer is **b**. Pain usually is not associated with the hair pulling by persons with this disorder. The DSM-IV definition of the disorder requires that the hair pulling result in noticeable hair loss. The most common areas affected are the eyebrows, the eyelashes, and the scalp, although any

area may be involved. Unlike the other Impulse-Control Disorders, the tension that usually precedes the act is absent, but tension is experienced when the individual attempts to resist the urge to pull hair. Males and females are equally represented among children, but in adults the disorder is more common in women. Some individuals may have the impulse to pull hair from others and from fibrous objects, such as carpets or sweaters. (*DSM-IV 618–621*)

65. Answer is **c**. The symptoms must develop within three months of the onset of the stressors and resolve within six months. However, DSM-IV has a qualifier of Chronic that allows for the persistence of symptoms past six months. The symptoms cannot represent Bereavement, since that is a separate diagnosis. Decreased work or school performance or a temporary change in social relationships would be typical of problems encountered in a person with a diagnosis of Adjustment Disorder. (*DSM-IV 623–627*)

66. Answer is **e**. A person's ethnicity, cultural background, and social situation must be considered in the evaluation for psychopathology. This is certainly true for the Personality Disorders, since many behaviors and traits may be culturally determined. By definition, a Personality Disorder puts the person in conflict with his or her culture. Diagnosis of Personality Disorders in a person under the age of 18 is possible only if the symptoms have been present for at least one year. Since the individual is in an active stage of development, care must be exercised before assigning a diagnosis of Personality Disorder. The exception is the Antisocial Personality Disorder, which can be diagnosed with some certainty before the age of 18. The development of significant personality changes beginning in middle adulthood or later requires a careful evaluation to ensure that a medical condition is not causing the changes. Some individuals may have a Personality Disorder become more evident when the person is under stress, such as with the loss of a job or the termination of a relationship. These losses may destabilize the individual and make the Personality Disorder more apparent. For those who have personality traits that are maladaptive or inflexible, but do not meet the criteria for a Personality Disorder, these maladaptive traits can be coded on Axis II. (*DSM-IV 629–634*)

67. Answer is **d**. Somewhat surprisingly, these individuals may form tightly knit groups that are centered around jointly held paranoid beliefs. Often they have thinly veiled fantasies of power or status that are unrealistic for them. Very brief psychotic episodes lasting minutes to hours can occur when the persons are stressed. However, if the individual is chronically psychotic, then the diagnosis would not be Paranoid Personality Disorder. Alcohol and Substance Abuse and Dependence are frequent problems associated with this diagnosis and in some cases the

diagnosis precedes the onset of Delusional Disorder or of Schizophrenia. (*DSM-IV 634–638*)

68. Answer is **a**. Paranoid ideation is frequently a part of the clinical picture, with these individuals often being suspicious of others. Their speech may be vague, digressive, or loose, but it is not incoherent and is without actual derailment. Dysphoric affects are frequently associated with this disorder. Anxiety and depression are common in this population, and 30–50% of those in a clinical setting will have a concurrent diagnosis of Major Depressive Disorder. Although the affective symptoms may be prominent, the hallmarks of the disorder are the cognitive and perceptual problems evident in these individuals. (*DSM-IV 641–642*)

69. Answer is **c**. While these individuals may be calculating in their exploitation of others, they can also display marked impulsivity and volatility. Rapid shifts in relationships, housing, and employment are highly characteristic of the disorder. A consistent disregard of the rights of others, with a pervasive pattern of the violation of their rights, is the essential feature of this disorder. The person must be 18 years of age or older, but some of the symptoms of the disorder must have been present before the age of 15. In many patients, the problems were apparent in childhood. Consistent and extreme irresponsibility is very characteristic of this disorder, and may involve all aspects of the individual's life. Lack of empathy, inflated self-appraisal, and superficial charm are characteristics classically associated with this disorder. (*DSM-IV 645–646*)

70. Answer is **e**. In their 30s and 40s, such persons may achieve the greatest degree of stability in vocational and interpersonal realms. The classic symptoms of this disorder are related to the individual's intense fear of real or imagined separation. Anxiety, despair, anger, and acting out may become manifest as the individual's fears are activated by external events. Most persons with this diagnosis are female. Complaints of emptiness, boredom, and a need to be occupied are frequent in this population. Attempted suicide is very common and 8–10% will die as a result of completed suicide. (*DSM-IV 650–654*)

71. Answer is **b**. The behavior of both men and women with this diagnosis tends to follow sex-role stereotype with men being excessively macho, whereas women may be hyperfeminized. These individuals are very suggestible and are easily influenced by prevailing trends. Delayed gratification is often met with angry outbursts. Their speech is highly impressionistic, imprecise, and lacking in detail or supporting facts. The actual prevalence of the disorder is unknown, but is probably about 2–3% of the general population and about 10–15 % in clinical settings. (*DSM-IV 655–656*)

72. Answer is **a**. Individuals with this diagnosis are very sensitive to the opinions of others and expect unqualified

admiration. The essential feature of the disorder is the pervasive pattern of grandiosity and lack of empathy that begins in early adulthood and is present in many contexts. These individuals are totally self-absorbed and frequently are insensitive to the feelings and needs of others. Their expectations are that others will be as absorbed with their welfare as they are, and they may be shocked and angered when the others are not. The unwillingness to take a risk or enter into a competitive situation may result in low vocational attainment. (*DSM-IV 658–659*)

73. Answer is **c**. These individuals have great difficulty expressing disagreement with those upon whom they depend. They are very reluctant to express even mild anger or hostility to those who are important to them. They allow others to take over their lives and to make important decisions for them. Feelings of incapability and an enduring need for help in almost every situation are all hallmarks of this disorder. Unfortunately, the perceived need for this level of emotional dependency often results in unbalanced and abusive relationships. This disorder is among the most frequently encountered Personality Disorders at mental health clinics. (*DSM-IV 666–667*)

74. Answer is **c**. The major neurotransmitter involved is believed to be acetylcholine, perhaps with lesser roles played by glutamate and serotonin. A number of brain structures are believed to be important in the genesis of delirium. The dorsal tegmental pathway and the reticular activating system are probably important in the mediation of delirium. Medications and combinations of medications are common causes of delirium, especially anticholinergic medications. (*SP 339*)

75. Answer is **c**. About half of patients with Dementia of the Alzheimer's Type experience their first symptoms between the ages of 65 and 70, although the disease can begin at any age. Transient ischemic attacks are brief periods of neurological dysfunction caused by microemboli, often originating in atherosclerotic plaques. About a third of patients with transient ischemic attacks will develop a subsequent brain infarction. The differentiation of pseudodementia from dementia is important and often difficult to accomplish. Patients with pseudodementia often complain more of cognitive problems than do patients with organically based dementia. Dementia due to HIV Disease has both a cognitive and a motoric component; this dementia frequently arises in end-stage AIDS. While a severe decline in memory or cognition is not a part of the normal aging process, minor memory problems are not uncommon. (*SP 354*)

76. Answer is **b**. The most commonly used illicit drug is cannabis, and 33% of the population have used it at some point in their lives. While cocaine and its derivatives are prominent in the media, cocaine is not the most frequently used illicit drug. The overwhelming majority of Amer-

icans have at least tried cigarettes and alcohol, although use of these two substances is declining. Forty percent of the population have tried an illicit substance. (*SP 387–388*)

77. Answer is **d**. A specific receptor for alcohol has not been identified. The benzodiazepines exert their action on the GABA receptor system. Cocaine exerts its clinical effects by enhancing the release of dopamine and norepinephrine. LSD attaches to the 5-HT$_2$ receptor. The cellular mechanism of alcohol has yet to be elucidated for its many and varied effects. (*SP 392*)

78. Answer is **d**. Episodes of violence may occur in individuals who have no previous history of violence, and users term such violence "roid rage". The episodes can involve murder, other violent acts. Adolescent boys frequently use the drugs to improve athletic performance and to enhance muscle development. About half of all users began their use before the age of 16. Significant mood alteration may be seen with maniclike symptoms occurring during periods of use and depression when off of the steroids. These drugs are classified in the same drug class as narcotics, Schedule III. Of special interest is the medical use of the available steroids to combat muscle wasting in certain medical conditions, such as malignancies and AIDS. Significant psychiatric sequelae can result in these patients as well. (*SP 394*)

79. Answer is **a**. The intoxicating effects of alcohol are greater when alcohol blood levels are rising then when they are falling. Most alcohol (90%) is absorbed by the small intestine, and its absorption is speeded up by drinking on an empty stomach. Ninety percent of alcohol is metabolized oxidatively by the liver at a constant rate, about 15 mg/dl/hr—the amount in a moderate sized drink. (*SP 400*)

80. Answer is **b**. Typically, these seizures occur in bursts, with the patient having more than one seizure in the three to six hours after the first seizure. The seizures are typical grand mal seizures with a generalized tonic-clonic characteristic patterns. Status epilepticus is rare in withdrawing alcoholics, and other causes of seizure activity must be investigated. Standard anticonvulsants should not be used in these patients as the seizure activity will cease when the withdrawal is treated. (*SP 404– 406*)

81. Answer is **e**. Autonomic hyperactivity is most common in these patients, with fever, diaphoresis, and hyperarousal being common features. The vivid, compelling hallucinations are a well-known component of the clinical picture. Typically, this syndrome will develop on the third hospital day, this being the third day of abstinence. Prompt recognition is important since untreated or undertreated DTs carries a high mortality rate. Benzodiazepines play a central role in the treatment of DTs and their prompt use can avert the development of this syndrome. (*SP 406– 407*)

82. Answer is **c**. Remote memory is preserved during a blackout, as are intellectual capabilities, and thus the patient may be able to perform complex tasks and to interact with others. Often the patient's behavior during a blackout is harmful or disturbing to others, and the patient may find reports about such behavior very disturbing. The patient will have no memory for a discrete period of time, much like the patient with transient global amnesia. Alcohol seems to block the incorporation of recent memories into remote memory. (*SP 407–408*)

83. Answer is **d**. Fluoxetine blocks the uptake of MDMA into the neuron and thus prevents its action, which is to cause a massive release of serotonin. The amphetamines are rapidly absorbed after oral administration. Classical amphetamines cause the release of norepinephrine and especially dopamine. The newer designer amphetamines also cause the release of serotonin. Serotonin has been implicated in the mediation of the hallucinatory activity of certain drugs of abuse. (*SP 412*)

84. Answer is **d**. Caffeine has many of the traits commonly associated with drugs of abuse. It is a positive reinforcer, especially at low doses. Humans and animals can distinguish caffeine from placebo in blinded conditions. Physical tolerance to some of the effects and withdrawal do occur. A cup of coffee contains about 100–150 mg of caffeine; tea contains about a third of that amount. The average adult in the United States consumes about 200 mg per day, and 20–39% consume more than 500 mg. Caffeine is a more potent xanthine than theophylline, the other commonly used methylxanthine. Three cups of coffee will contain enough caffeine to occupy 50% of all adenosine receptors in the brain. Effects on dopamine and norepinephrine are also part of caffeine's action. (*SP 416–417*)

85. Answer is **c**. Animals do not self-administer cannabis as they do with the other drugs of abuse. This drug is used mostly by young adults and adolescents. A specific receptor has been identified and is found in highest concentrations in the basal ganglia, the hippocampus, and the cerebellum. Only a limited withdrawal is noted in humans, with some symptoms of activation, such as restlessness and insomnia, noted. The classic signs of cannabis intoxication are injected conjunctiva, mild tachycardia, dry mouth, and the well-known appetite stimulation. (*SP 420–422*)

86. Answer is **c**. Cocaine is a central nervous system stimulant and results in activation of the person using it. Seizures associated with cocaine use are usually solitary, but may be multiple. Myocardial infarction and death are often associated with use of this drug. Patients who inhale powdered cocaine may sustain significant damage to the mucosal lining of the nose. Nonhemorrhagic cerebral infarction is the most common cerebrovascular disease associated with cocaine use. (*SP 426*)

87. Answer is **e**. Cocaine is a powerfully addicting substance associated with an unpleasant withdrawal. Often the patient will deny the need for treatment in spite of serious consequences associated with continued use. Resistance to treatment is common in these individuals, and random drug screens are often necessary to ensure abstinence. The clinician should be aware of the intense craving for the drug in the early phases of withdrawal, and may have to hospitalize the patient to remove him or her from contact with drugs and drug-related activity. (*SP 425–429*)

88. Answer is **b**. White males are twice as likely as black males to be users of hallucinogens. Users of these drugs are more likely to live in the western United States and to be age 15–35 years. Hallucinogen use is associated with much lower mortality and morbidity, and only 1% of emergency room visits are associated with these drugs. As the drug users of the 1960s have aged, the lifetime rates of hallucinogen use by older adults have steadily increased from 1974 to the present. (*SP 430–443*)

89. Answer is **b**. Use of alcohol and the inhalants simultaneously increases the intoxicating effects of the inhalant, probably owing to competition for hepatic enzymes. Inhalants produce a sense of euphoria or excitement in users, but usually are used for only a short time because the user moves on to other drugs of abuse or stops drug use. Most of the inhalants are metabolized by the liver, with a small amount being excreted by the lungs. Long-term use of organic solvents can result in serious neurological problems, including decreased intelligence, brain atrophy, and temporal lobe epilepsy. (*SP 433–437*)

90. Answer is **d**. Nicotine is a highly addicting and toxic substance. Doses of 60 mg will kill an adult human by respiratory paralysis. Cigarettes deliver about 0.5 mg. Smoking rates in the psychiatric population are much higher than in the general population, and smoking is almost universal among patients with Schizophrenia. Nicotine has complex effects on the central nervous system and may exert its addicting influence by stimulation of the dopaminergic projections from the ventral tegmental area to the cortex and the limbic system. The costs associated with tobacco use are astronomical, with 60% of direct health care costs attributed to its use and the resultant illnesses, or about $1 billion a day. (*SP 436–438*)

91. Answer is **e**. Codeine is transformed into morphine in the body. Specific receptors for the opiates have been known for almost 20 years. The ventral tegmental area plays a central role in the addiction process. Opiates have complex effects on the dopaminergic and noradrenergic systems in the body. Heroin is more potent than morphine, is more lipid soluble, and has a more rapid onset of action. (*SP 439–440*)

92. Answer is **d**. The cause of death from an opioid overdose is almost always respiratory depression, not cardiac arrest. Tolerance to the opioids develops rapidly, and withdrawal to morphine and heroin develops only six to eight hours after the last dose. Typical withdrawal symptoms include gastrointestinal distress, rhinorrhea, lacrimation, and yawning. The withdrawal syndrome can be acutely produced by the opioid antagonists, which exert their effects immediately after administration. (*SP 443– 444*)

93. Answer is **d**. Individuals may become tolerant to the effects of PCP, but do not develop physical dependence. Originally PCP was developed as an anesthetic, but its use was discontinued when patients awoke with unpleasant hallucinations, disorientation, agitation, and delirium. Ketamine is an anesthetic used in humans that is chemically related to PCP, but lacks its unpleasant effects, and it also is subject to abuse. PCP binds to the NMDA receptor and prevents the influx of calcium ions. It also stimulates the dopaminergic neurons of the ventral tegmental area, a key factor in its abuse potential. The highest rate of use is in the Washington, D.C. area, with PCP accounting for 18% of substance–related deaths. (*SP 447– 449*)

94. Answer is **c**. Talking down, a technique commonly used in the management of patients who have taken hallucinogens, is not effective in the acute management of PCP. Benzodiazepines are often the drug of choice in the management of the behavioral disturbances that are manifest in these patients. Hypertension is common and may require treatment. Use of four-point restraints is a dangerous technique because it may lead to rhabdomylinosis. Acidification of the urine will speed the excretion of the drug. (*SP 449– 450*)

95. Answer is **b**. Severe seizures, including status epilepticus, may take place during withdrawal from the barbiturates, and death may result. The withdrawal from alcohol also has significant morbidity and mortality, but they are not as high as from barbiturates. The same is true of the benzodiazepines. Withdrawal from the opioids and the hallucinogens is usually not associated with the risk of death. (*SP 454– 455*)

96. Answer is **b**. Schizophrenic patients who smoke are less likely to have drug–induced parkinsonism due to the nicotine-induced activation of the dopaminergic neurons. The seasonality of birth as it relates to the schizophrenic population is well known, although its significance is unknown. Individuals with Schizophrenia tend to die at earlier ages than the general population from both accidents and natural causes. Fifty percent of schizophrenic patients will attempt suicide, and 10–15% will die as a result of suicide. The fertility rate for schizophrenic patient is almost that of the general population owing to the advances in pharmacotherapy, the emphasis on reha-

bilitation, and a general increase in the rates of marriage and fertility these individuals. (*SP 461– 462*)

97. Answer is **b**. Clozapine is an effective antipsychotic and its effect on the $D_2$ receptor is minimal. It also has activity in the serotonin system, and the role of serotonin in the pathogenesis of Schizophrenia is being actively investigated. At its most fundamental level, the dopamine hypothesis states that schizophrenic individuals exhibit an overactivity of the dopaminergic system; the role of other neurotransmitters is being actively investigated. Serotonin may play a role in the impulsive and suicidal behaviors so frequently seen in these patients. Elevated plasma levels of dopamine's major metabolite, homovanillic acid, have been well established in schizophrenic patients, and when treated with antipsychotic medications, these levels fall. Advances in imaging technology have resulted in a series of studies that have revealed ventricular enlargement and a reduced brain volume. (*SP 464– 466*)

98. Answer is **b**. Olfactory and gustatory hallucinations are uncommon, and their presence requires a careful evaluation to rule out the presence of a medical or neurological disorder. An illusion is the misinterpretation of a real environmental stimulus; a hallucination is a sensory experience in the absence of environmental stimuli. Hearing two or more voices engaged in a running commentary about the patient's behavior is a common experience among schizophrenic patients. A cenesthetic hallucination is the experience of a bodily sensation that is unfounded or is impossible to experience. (*SP 477*)

99. Answer is **a**. Males with Schizophrenia are more likely to commit suicide than are females. Youth and education increase the risk of suicide, as does living alone and a change in the course of illness. Since 50% of schizophrenic individuals attempt suicide and 10–15% die as a result, careful assessment of the risk factors is essential. (*SP 462*)

100. Answer is **b**. Postpartum Psychosis is a psychiatric emergency and most often will require hospitalization. Carefully supervised visits with the infant may be possible, but an affected woman should not be allowed to care for the infant without supervision. Infanticide is a major concern. The majority of women with this disorder have just had their first child, and 50% of affected individuals have had nonpsychiatric perinatal complications. Relatives of affected women have an incidence of Mood Disorders similar to that of persons with Mood Disorders. Postpartum Psychosis may be viewed as a Mood Disorder, and use of an antidepressant and lithium may be the treatment of choice. However, treatment with antipsychotic medications may be indicated. (*SP 494– 495*)

101. Answer is **d**. Delusional Disorders can be treated in an outpatient setting, but after a complete inpatient evalua-

tion. These are very difficult patients in terms of treatment. For a positive outcome, the therapist must be able to penetrate the patient's basic mistrust; delusions must be diminished, and social adjustment is required. (*SP 510–512*)

**102–105.** Answers are: 102 **d**; 103 **a**; 104 **c**; and 105 **b**. The chief characteristic of the autoscopic psychosis is the experiencing of a visual hallucination of a part of one's body. Amok is characterized by the person's suddenly developing an attack of wild rage. Affected individuals require physical restraint until the attack passes. Capgras's syndrome is characterized by the delusion that persons close to the patient have been replaced by impostors. This delusion may occur in an otherwise clear sensorium. Cotard's syndrome, also known as Nihilistic Delusional Disorder, is characterized by the delusion that one has lost everything, including one's own internal organs, and that the world beyond the patient is reduced to nothingness. (*SP 492–493*)

**106.** Answer is **B**. Individuals with the diagnosis of Gender Identity Disorder have a characteristic pattern of cross—gender identification and a persistent discomfort with the assigned sex. As an adult, the individual may focus on the issue of gender distress, and his or her activities may revolve around this issue. These individuals are not homosexual, although they choose sexual partners of the same sex. The basis for the choice of same-sex partner is the feeling that the person is not a member of the assigned sex, but rather of the other sex, and thus chooses a partner from a heterosexual viewpoint. Most homosexuals are not distressed by their assigned sex and do not have a desire to be the other sex. As children, these individuals may not adhere to the behavior expected of the assigned sex, but actively participate in activities most associated with the other sex, and thus encounter strong disapproval from parents and society. (*DSM-IV 532–537*)

**107.** Answer is **C**. Snacking all day would not constitute a binge. A binge is the eating of an amount of food that is in excess of the amount that would be ordinarily consumed in a given period. Binges frequently have triggers, such as dysphoric mood states, interpersonal stressors, or intense hunger. Self–induced vomiting is the most common compensatory mechanism for the overconsumption of food. Rarely, an emetic, a laxative, or an enema will be employed as a means of compensating for a binge. (*DSM-IV 545–547*)

**108.** Answer is **E**. The most common complaints are of difficulty in falling asleep or in maintaining sleep; less commonly, the individual may complain only of poor-quality sleep or of nonrestorative sleep. Frequently, these individuals may have a lifelong history of poor sleep. This tendency may have a familial tendency. Complaints of insomnia increase with age and are more common in women. (*DSM-IV 553–556*)

**109.** Answer is **C**. Males are affected three times more frequently than are females. Symptoms of disinhibition may be seen between periods of excessive sleepiness and include hypersexuality and inappropriate sexual advances. Compulsive overeating with weight gain may also be a symptom. (*DSM-IV 558*)

**110.** Answer is **A**. First-degree relatives of individuals with Narcolepsy have a high rate of disorders of excessive sleepiness, and a multifactorial mode of inheritance seems to be the route of genetic transmission. The daytime sleepiness is stable over time and generally is the first symptom to appear, usually in adolescence. The male-to-female ratio is 1:1.(*DSM-IV 562–566*)

**111.** Answer is **D**. Obstructive sleep apnea syndrome is the most common type of sleep apnea. Periods of breathing cessation can last up to 90 seconds and are frequently associated with the development of cyanosis. Most individuals are not aware of their problem, and their bed partners are the ones who insist on evaluation of the very loud snoring associated with the breathing stoppage. (*DSM-IV 568*)

**112.** Answer is **A**. Central sleep apnea involves the cessation of breathing due to a cessation of respiratory effort. The origin of this disorder is in the central nervous system and is not associated with airway obstruction. Central alveolar hypoventilation syndrome is a condition of already compromised arterial oxygen levels that is aggravated by sleep. This condition is seen mostly in very overweight persons. All of the sleep apneas are more common in older populations, and some elderly individuals may experience ventilation problems because of neurological or vascular problems. The male-to-female ratio for obstructive sleep apnea is 8:1. (*DSM-IV 570–571*)

**113.** Answer is **C**. Injury can readily occur during a sleepwalking episode since the individual is not truly aware of the environment, and may fall out of windows or walk into traffic. Usually the behaviors are of low complexity and of a routine nature, but more complex behaviors can be observed. Occasionally, the patient may speak or operate equipment, but this is the exception rather than the rule. Like the Sleep Terror Disorder, the Sleepwalking Disorder does not take place during REM sleep, but during stages 3 and 4. Sleepwalking can occur whenever an individual is capable of walking, but the first episode typically is seen between the ages of 4 and 8 and the disorder spontaneously remits during adolescence. New-onset sleepwalking in adults is rare and should be carefully evaluated to rule out other causes, such as substance abuse. (*DSM-IV 588–588*)

**114.** Answer is **A**. Only about 5% of all shoplifters have this diagnosis, and it is more common in women. These individuals know that the act of stealing is senseless and wrong, and most could have easily afforded the item stolen. Although the acts of stealing are not planned, the individual fears negative repercussions. By definition, these acts of stealing are not acts motivated by anger or revenge, nor are they based on delusional material. (*DSM-IV 612–613*)

115. Answer is **E**. Pathological gamblers are often seeking "action" as much as they are seeking money, and will often play for ever-higher stakes to achieve a certain level of excitement. This frequently results in a pattern of "chasing" losses by increasing bets in a vain attempt to make up for lost funds. About one third of all individuals with this diagnosis are females, though less than 5% of the membership of Gamblers Anonymous are women, probably because of the greater stigma associated with this problem for females. Alcohol Dependence and Pathological Gambling are more common in the parents of individuals with the diagnosis of Pathological Gambling than in the general population. Individuals with this diagnosis are often energetic, competitive, and easily bored. They may be excessively generous to the point of extravagance. (*DSM-IV 615–617*)

116. Answer is **A**. The key to the diagnosis of any Personality Disorder is a long-standing pattern of maladaptive and inflexible personality traits that interfere with interpersonal relationships and occupational functioning. The clinician must establish, through careful evaluation, that these traits have been present since early adulthood or adolescence. The traits are pervasive and are manifest in all aspects of the patient's life. A complicating factor in the establishment of the diagnosis is the ego syntonicity of many of the traits and patterns. The individual with this diagnosis may not have a sense of inner turmoil and pain, but others may experience distress when interacting with the individual. (*DSM-IV 630–632*)

117. Answer is **D**. Individuals with this disorder have a general distrust of others, including those whom they know well. The behaviors of friends and family are closely scrutinized for evidence of hostile intentions. Spouses and significant others may be suspected of being unfaithful, without justification. These individuals can be very difficult to get along with in all situations. They may complain incessantly and be argumentative. They often hold grudges and are unwilling to forgive others for perceived insults and injuries. (*DSM-IV 634–636*)

118. Answer is **D**. Individuals with this disorder are insensitive to what others think of them and are indifferent to criticism. They are cold and aloof and generally display little affect. The expression of anger may be especially difficult for these individuals. They seem to derive little pleasure from any relationships, including with the family of origin. They have a sole confidant, but are often without any relationships at all. This disorder appears to be more common in males, although it is an uncommon disorder. (*DSM-IV 638–639*)

119. Answer is **E**. Individuals with this diagnosis are often tense, easily bored, and depressed. The prevalence among males is 3% and in females about 1%. Some concern has been expressed about its underdiagnosis in females due to the emphasis on aggressive aspects of the individual's behavior. This disorder appears to be associated with lower socioeconomic status and urban life. First-degree biological relatives of individuals have an increased rate of Substance Abuse Disorder and Somatization Disorder. (*DSM-IV 645–650*)

120. Answer is **A**. Fears of rejection, criticism, and embarrassment prevent these individuals from engaging in normal social and occupational activities. Strong feelings of inferiority and low self-esteem also play roles in the inhibited lives of these people. They have equally strong desires for love from and acceptance by others. The pattern of shyness and social inhibition frequently begins in infancy and becomes a lifelong pattern of interpersonal interaction. (*DSM-IV 662–663*)

121. Answer is **C**. Individuals with this disorder are as ruthless and merciless concerning their own performance as they are about the shortcomings of others. They are rigid and inflexible in their behavior and thinking. Decisions are slowly arrived at, if ever, for fear of making the wrong decision and thus decisions are delayed ever longer as more data are accumulated to support the "right" decision. These individuals are always expecting a disaster in the future, and thus live far below their incomes in order to prepare for the future disaster. (*DSM-IV 669–671*)

122. Answer is **A**. The distribution of pathological changes in the brain differs with the type of pathological process present. Dementia of the Alzheimer's Type affects the parietal-temporal areas of the brain and the Pick's Disease affects the frontotemporal regions. Vascular dementia, called multi-infarct dementia in DSM-III-R, is more common in men and is characterized by multiple infarcts of the brain. Patients with a history of hypertension are most prone to the development of this type of dementia. Binswanger's disease is also known as subcortical arteriosclerotic encephalopathy, and is characterized by the presence of many small infarctions of the white matter. It may be more common than was previously thought. (*SP 345–347*)

123. Answer is **E**. Chronic alcoholism is the classic condition associated with Korsakoff's syndrome. A deficiency of thiamine is the cause of the syndrome, and other conditions that cause nutritional compromise may result in this disorder. Confabulation is most often associated with this disorder, although apathy and passivity may be associated with it as well. (*SP 359*)

124. Answer is **E**. The HIV-infected patient brings a host of issues to the psychotherapeutic situation. Health care decisions should be fully explored and should include

issues regarding terminal care and life support. Engaging the patient in these discussions will keep the locus of control with the patient and avoid hurried decisions in a crisis situation. Substance use and abuse should be extensively reviewed with the patient, since these can contribute substantially to the patient's morbidity and mortality. (*SP 381–382*)

125. Answer is **B**. Comorbidity is the presence of two or more psychiatric diagnoses in a single patient. Men with Substance Abuse or Dependence Disorders have a 75% chance of having a comorbid condition and women have a 65% chance. The most frequent comorbid condition is the Antisocial Personality Disorder. In general, the more potent and dangerous the substance the greater is the risk of a comorbid condition. (*SP 389–390*)

126. Answer is **A**. Psychodynamic theories posit oral anxiety as potentially causative, with the consumption of alcohol being anxiolytic. Mounting evidence points to the heritability of the vulnerability to develop Alcohol-Related Disorders, with individuals having first-degree relatives with Alcohol-Related Disorders having a three-fold to four-fold greater risk of developing alcoholism than those who do not have first-degree relatives who are alcoholic. Certain environments tolerate, and indeed may encourage, the overuse and abuse of alcohol. While family attitudes and the use of alcohol play a role in the behavior of children with regard to alcohol, they are not as great an influence as was once thought. (*SP 399*)

127. Answer is **B**. Wernicke's Syndrome may progress to Korsakoff's syndrome if untreated, not vice versa. Ataxia with a gait disturbance is common in these patients, as are bilateral eye findings. The eye findings may not be symmetrical, but they are bilateral. (*SP 407*)

128. Answer is **E**. Fetal Alcohol Syndrome is a common and complex syndrome with both anatomical abnormalities and many maladaptive behaviors of the individuals as adolescents and adults. This syndrome is the leading cause of mental retardation in the United States and the chance of an alcoholic woman's having a defective child is 35%. (*SP 409*)

129. Answer is **C**. There are striking similarities between the Amphetamine-Induced Psychosis and Paranoid Schizophrenia. Both have paranoid ideation as a hallmark symptom and at times are clinically indistinguishable. The patient with an Amphetamine-Induced Psychosis tends to have more prominent visual hallucinations and, be more hyperactive and hypersexual. (*SP 413–414*)

130. Answer is **E**. Almost 20% of adults ages 18 to 26 reported having tried cocaine at least once in their lifetimes, and more than a third of adults ages 26 to 34 reported the same. Lifetime use of cocaine in adults age 26 and older

is steadily climbing. Males are twice as likely as females to have tried cocaine in the previous month. While the West showed slightly higher use rates, use across the regions of the United States did not vary at statistically significant levels. (*SP 423–424*)

131. Answer is **D**. Heroin is the most commonly used opioid among abusers. Males are three times more likely than females to be opioid users. There are about a half a million opioid users in the United States, with about half of them living in New York City. The use of dirty needles by opioid addicts and unprotected sex have played a major role in the transmission of HIV. (*SP 439– 440*)

132. Answer is **E**. The validity of the prodromal symptoms has been questioned because these symptoms and signs are almost always diagnosed in retrospect and thus are contaminated by the clinician's awareness of the full-blown syndrome. Friends and family may note a decreased level of occupational and/or social functioning, usually described as the patient's not being himself or herself. Often the premorbid history of the schizophrenic individual is one of passivity, aloofness, and shyness, with new interests in the abstract or occult developing in the premorbid phase. (*SP 476*)

133. Answer is **A**. An effective link between the schizophrenic patient and available community services is an important goal of hospitalization. This can prevent relapses and enhance the person's quality of life. The hospital provides a respite from the demands of independent living, and can help the patient regain the skills of daily living. Typical indications for hospitalization include suicidal acts or thoughts, grossly disorganized behavior, and medication stabilization. Shorter term hospitalization (six weeks or less) with an active, behaviorally oriented therapeutic approach has proved to be more effective than a longer-term hospitalization with a custodial or insight-oriented approach. (*SP 481*)

134. Answer is **E**. The initial step in the treatment of this disorder is the separation of the partners. All affected individuals must receive some type of treatment, and frequently that involves psychotherapy. The dominant partner must be carefully diagnoses and treated. Increasing the contact of the affected individuals with the outside world may be helpful in preventing a relapse. (*SP 492*)

135. Answer is **A**. A fluctuating level of consciousness is very characteristic of delirium and differentiates it from dementia and other processes. Disturbances in the sleep wake cycle are common and prominent, with the patient's, occasionally having day–night reversal. The EEG is usually abnormal, showing either generalized slowing or fast activity. (*DSM-IV 124–126*)

136. Answer is **C**. DSM-IV abandons the term "organic mental disorder" stating that it implies that other disorders

lack a biological basis. Dementia, Delirium, Amnestic Disorders, and other cognitive disorders are grouped together in DSM-IV. DSM-IV has separate categories for Substance Abuse disorders, but does have categories for dementia and delirium caused by substances. DSM-IV has categories for "Dementia Due to . . . ." and the etiology, if known, is added. For example, Dementia Due to Pick's Disease would be a DSM-IV diagnosis. (*DSM-IV 139–155*)

137. Answer is **E**. Patients with Substance Dependence continue to use substances even in the face of serious consequences. Their social and occupational functioning is impaired by their continued use and abuse of substances. According to DSM-IV, Substance Dependence as a diagnosis applies to many substances, except for caffeine. The need for ever-greater amounts of a substance to achieve intoxication or the desired effect is the hallmark of Substance Dependence. Some substances, (e.g., cannabis) do not result in withdrawal or tolerance, yet some individuals exhibit compulsive use patterns. Substance Dependence is more than physiological; it invokes the cognitive and behavioral patterns of the individual in its definition. (*DSM-IV 176–178*)

138. Answer is **C**. The specifiers in DSM-IV are attempts to characterize the various subtypes of remission observed in patients following a period of substance use. DSM-IV sets the period of one month since the period of dependence as the time frame for the use of specifiers. The first 12 months following Dependence are designated Early Remission, and if the patient suffers a relapse without a return to the full criteria for Dependence, then the specifier is Early Partial Remission. Sustained Full Remission takes a number of factors into account: the length of time of Dependence, the duration of non-use, and the need for continued monitoring and evaluation. The Sustained Full Remission Specifier could begin after the first 12 months since the period of Dependence, if no criteria for Dependence are met during that initial 12 months. (*DSM-IV 279–283*)

139. Answer is **E**. The diagnosis of Schizophrenia is a composite of a number of signs and symptoms and no single sign or symptom is pathognomonic for Schizophrenia. Positive symptoms reflect exaggeration or distortions of normal function (e.g., hallucinations) and negative symptoms reflect a diminution of normal function. Patients who experience general and nonspecific environmental cues, such as advertisements having a special and specific meaning directed at them, are experiencing referential delusions. The time boundaries set by DSM-IV for Schizophrenia symptomatology are one month in which signs and symptoms are strongly present and six months of some evidence of the disorder. Isolated episodes of symptoms do not meet criteria for Schizophrenia. (*DSM-IV 273–278*)

140. Answer is **A**. DSM-IV includes affective flattening, alogia, and avolition as its criteria for diagnosis, however, anhedonia is included in the "associated features and disorders" section. Negative symptoms are almost ubiquitous in Schizophrenia, although they may be difficult to specify. Undesirable side effects of neuroleptics include extrapyramidal side effects that can mimic avolition or alogia. (*DSM-IV 277*)

141. Answer is **B**. The educational process for young individuals with Schizophrenia may be severely disrupted by the development of the disorder. Individuals with Schizophrenia are frequently unemployed or underemployed, the so-called "downward drift" of Schizophrenia. The majority (60–70%) of such persons do not marry and are socially isolated. DSM-IV requires an active phase of at least one month in duration and significant symptoms that persist for six months. Negative symptoms are quite common in both the prodromal and residual phases. (*DSM-IV 279–283*)

142. Answer is **D**. The course of Schizophrenia can be quite variable, with some individuals displaying exacerbations and remissions, whereas others remain chronically ill. Negative symptoms may become more prominent as the illness progresses. Acute onset, good premorbid adjustment, later age at onset, being female, and associated mood disturbance all predict a better prognosis. Men tend to have a first psychotic episode in their early to mid-20s, or when slightly younger than women whose first episode tends to occur in the late 20s. (*DSM-IV 282*)

143. Answer is **E**. The Disorganized Type of Schizophrenia is probably the most severe form, often following a course that shows no significant remissions. Speech and behavior are severely disorganized, resulting in profound problems for these patients. Activities of daily living may be severely impaired, and a supervised environment may be required. The affects expressed by these patients are often incongruous with the thoughts expressed and may often be marked by silliness or laughter out of context. (*DSM-IV 287–288*)

144. Answer is **E**. The diagnostic criteria for Schizophrenia and Schizophreniform Disorder are identical except for two differences. First, the symptomatology of Schizophreniform Disorder is limited to six months. If the symptoms persist beyond six months, the diagnosis of Schizophrenia applies. Second, impairment of social or occupational functioning is not required for a diagnosis of Schizophreniform Disorder. The diagnosis of Schizophreniform Disorder does not exclude psychotic features. (*DSM-IV 290–291*)

145. Answer is **A**. For a diagnosis of Schizoaffective Disorder, symptoms of both Schizophrenia and a Mood Disorder must coexist during a significant portion of the total dura-

tion of the illness. Specifically, symptoms must meet the criteria for Major Depressive, Manic, or Mixed Episode and Schizophrenia, Criterion A. Merely having a brief episode of Mood Disorder in the midst of a process of Schizophrenia of long duration would not meet the criteria for Schizoaffective Disorder. (*DSM-IV 291–293*)

146. Answer is **C**. As defined by DSM-IV, the Brief Psychotic Disorder (Brief Reactive Psychosis in DSM-III-R) lasts at least one day, but not longer than one month. If symptoms persist longer than one month, then Schizophreniform Disorder would apply. Emotional turmoil with rapid affective shifts is often seen with this disorder. An especially high suicide risk in younger patients with this diagnosis has been observed. By definition, this disorder resolves completely and the individual returns to premorbid level of functioning. (*DSM-IV 302–303*)

147. Answer is **D**. This disorder is not a psychological reaction to having a medical condition, but rather the medical condition causes the psychosis. Brain lesions or insults are frequent causes of this diagnosis and hallucinatory phenomena in all sensory modalities, as well as delusions, are common. The essential feature of this diagnosis is that the psychosis is the result of a medical condition. (*DSM-IV 307–308*)

148. Answer is **E**. For this diagnosis, the criteria for both Manic Episode and Major Depressive Episode nearly every day for one week must be met. The patient experiences rapidly alternating moods in conjunction with the symptoms of a Manic Episode and a Major Depressive Episode. Agitation, insomnia, appetite deregulation, psychotic features, and suicidal ideation are frequently seen in this clinical situation. Evidence is accumulating that some patients have a bipolar "diathesis" that results in Mixed-like Episodes following somatic treatment for depression (antidepressants, light therapy, etc.). Younger patients and those over 60 with Bipolar Disorder seem especially prone to developing Mixed Episodes. Males may be more affected than females by this disorder. (*DSM-IV 333*)

149. Answer is **A**. Major Depressive Disorders have one or more Major Depressive Episodes but never a Manic Episode, a Hypomanic Episode, or a Mixed Episode. DSM-IV has four specifiers for severity and seven for the status of the disorder. Severity specifiers are Mild, Moderate, and Severe With Psychotic Features. The status of the disorder is indicated by the specifiers of In Partial Remission or In Full Remission, or Chronic With Catatonic Features, With Melancholic Features, With Atypical Features, and With Postpartum Onset. For a particular episode to be considered to have ended, the full criteria for the Major Depressive Episode, must have not been met for two months. (*DSM-IV 339–341*)

150. Answer is **D**. Typically, the first Major Depressive Episode is in the mid-20s, however, it can occur any time in life. Some 50%–60% of individuals with Major Depressive Disorder, Single Episode, can be expected to have a second episode, and those with two episodes have a 70% chance of having a third. Patients with three episodes have a 90% chance of having a fourth episode. Remissions tend to be longer earlier in the course of illness and shorter later in the course. Of individuals with Major Depressive Disorder, Single Episode, 5% to 10% go on to develop Bipolar I disorder. (*DSM-IV 341*)

151. Answer is **B**. Some 25% to 50% of patients with Dysthymic Disorder will have some of the same findings on polysomnography that are seen in individuals with Major Depressive Disorder. In adulthood, women are two to three times more likely to develop Dysthymic Disorder than are men. The severity of symptoms and the presence of pronounced vegetative symptoms are important in the differentiation of Dysthymic Disorder from Major Depressive Disorder. Chronic mood disturbance, especially depressive symptoms, are quite common in Axis II disorders, and thus Dysthymic Disorder is frequently associated with the Personality Disorders. (*DSM-IV 346*)

152. Answer is **A**. Bipolar I Disorder includes a Manic or Mixed Episode as a part of the diagnosis, whereas Bipolar II Disorder has Hypomanic Episodes as part of the diagnosis. Recent studies indicate that Bipolar I Disorder occurs equally in men and women, while women are heavily represented in Bipolar II Disorder populations. Psychotic symptoms are less frequent in all phases of Bipolar II Disorder; both depressive and hypomanic Bipolar I Disorder more frequently result in psychotic features of the disorder. (*DSM-IV 352–356*)

153. Answer is **D**. Community studies indicate that the lifetime prevalence of Bipolar II Disorder is about 0.5%. With increasing age, the intervals between episodes tend to decrease, resulting in a greater management challenge for both patient and psychiatrist. A majority of individuals return to full function between episodes, with about 15% retaining significant symptoms. Over five years, 5–15% of individuals develop a Manic Episode, and thus would be rediagnosed as having Bipolar I Disorder. (*DSM-IV 360–361*)

154. Answer is **B**. The Mood Disorders specifier With Melancholic Features applies to severely depressed individuals who have lost all or almost all responsivity to pleasurable stimuli. The individual remains depressed, with little or no affective brightening in response to positive circumstances or events. These individuals have early-morning awakening, depression that is worse in morning, and a marked psychomotor disturbance. Affected individuals are less likely to have a preexisting Personality Disorder, a clear precipitant, or a significant

placebo response. These severely depressed individuals frequently require hospitalization. (*DSM-IV 383*)

155. Answer is **E**. When using the Longitudinal Course Specifiers for Mood Disorders, the two most recent episodes should be evaluated. The pattern associated with the best prognosis is a Major Depressive Disorder without antecedent Dysthymic Disorder and a complete remission of symptoms between episodes. The presence of Dysthymic Disorder before the onset of Major Depressive Disorder with incomplete resolution of symptoms between episodes correlates with the poorest prognosis. This pattern of Dysthymic Disorder coupled with Major Depressive Disorder has been called the "double depression." These same specifiers can be applied to the Bipolar I Disorder and Bipolar II Disorder and to characterize the presence or absence of mood symptoms between episodes. (*DSM-IV 389*)

156. Answer is **D**. Usually Rapid Cycling is associated with a poor outcome. DSM-IV sets 4 or more episodes of mood switches in one year as the number needed to meet the criteria. The episodes must meet the criteria for Major Depressive, Mixed or Manic, and a period of no symptoms must intervene or there is a switch from one pole to its opposite. The episodes are exactly like Major Depressive, Manic or Mixed, but occur with greater rapidity. Although Bipolar Disorder has an equal sex ratio, women account for 70–90% of individuals with a Rapid Cycling pattern. Although more frequently diagnosed in women, to meet the criteria for this specifier the episodes cannot be linked to phases of the menstrual cycle. (*DSM-IV 390*)

157. Answer is **C**. Agoraphobia is not a codable diagnosis in DSM-IV. DSM-IV sets criteria for Agoraphobia to clarify what is meant by the term. The essential feature of Agoraphobia is anxiety about being in a situation from which escape could be difficult or embarrassing or in which help may not be available in the event a situation-bound or an unexpected Panic Attack occurs. Typically, individuals with Agoraphobia avoid situations that may cause anxiety, and they are never alone. This behavior may severely limit their social and/or occupational function or a relationship may be severely strained by the insistence of the patient on not being alone. Agoraphobia should not be diagnosed if the anxiety or phobic avoidance can be better accounted for by another disorder. (*DSM-IV 396–398*)

158. Answer is **B**. The focus of the fear is important in this differential. Many patients with Panic Disorder have unexpected Panic Attacks and tend to focus their anxiety on the recurrence of Panic Attacks rather than on a specific situation or external stimulus. Panic Disorder With Agoraphobia would be associated with unexpected Panic Attacks and would have more frequent attacks than with Panic Disorder alone. Also, since the fears of the individual with Panic Disorder With Agoraphobia are less specific than in Specific Phobia, Situational Type, the patient with Panic Disorder With Agoraphobia will avoid situations in general. For example, an individual with Panic Disorder with Agoraphobia might avoid all situations where he or she might be alone, whereas the individual with Specific Phobia, Situational Type, will avoid specific situations, such as flying in airplanes. (*DSM-IV 401*)

159. Answer is **A**. Women are much more frequently diagnosed with this disorder than are men. Cultural influences may play a role in the greater representation of females in the diagnostic category. Individuals with this disorder have never met the criteria for Panic Disorder, and the focus of their fear is not on having full-blown Panic Attacks but rather on having Partial Attacks. Panic Disorder With Agoraphobia is far more commonly diagnosed in clinical samples than is Agoraphobia Without History of Panic Disorder. (*DSM-IV 403–404*)

160. Answer **E**. Women account for most of the cases of Specific Phobia. For example, approximately 75–90% of Specific Phobia, Situational Type, are women. Most types of Specific Phobia have origins in childhood, although true new-onset Situational Type can occur in early adulthood. This accounts for the bimodal age of onset for the Situational Type of one peak in childhood and another in early adulthood. Fears of blood and injury may have especially strong familial patterns. (*DSM-IV 408–409*)

161. Answer is **C**. This diagnosis occurs equally in males and females. According to DSM-IV, adults with the disorder must realize the unreasonable nature of their obsessions and compulsions at some time during the course of illness. This is not true for children, however. Individuals with this disorder typically avoid situations that involve the context of their obsessions. For example, obsessions about dirt or contamination may lead to an avoidance of using public rest rooms, shaking hands, handling money, etc. This avoidance may severely affect the person's social and occupational functions. Tourette's Disorder has Obsessive-Compulsive Disorder as an additional associated feature 35–50% of the time. However, the incidence of Tourette's Disorder in Obsessive-Compulsive Disorder is only 5–7%, although 20–30% of individuals with the latter disorder may report having current or past tics. (*DSM-IV 417–420*)

162. Answer is **E**. The "psychic numbness" or "emotional anesthesia" represents a decreased responsiveness to the external world, and previously enjoyed activities are greeted with disinterest. Affected individuals may also feel persistent arousal or anxiety that is new for them, and feel they have no future. Career plans, marriage, and other long-term situations may seem improbable or unlikely. The severity, duration, and proximity of the trauma may

be important factors in determining the development of this disorder. Daily experiences of severe trauma, such as being in a concentration camp, may produce this disorder more often more often than would a single, brief traumatic event. However, individual vulnerability will vary, and thus will the development of this disorder in response to a traumatic event. (*DSM-IV 425–426*)

163. Answer is **B**. Two major differences separate these diagnoses. First, Acute Stress Disorder has an onset shortly after the traumatic experience and ends within four weeks. PTSD may have quite a delayed onset of symptoms and an indefinite course of illness. Second, the DSM-IV criteria emphasizes the role of dissociative symptoms in patients with Acute Stress Disorder. While either diagnosis may have dissociative symptoms as a feature, the diagnosis of Acute Stress Disorder has such symptoms as a prominent feature. The severity of the trauma is not a differentiating criterion and individuals with Acute Stress Disorder frequently reexperience the traumatic event just as those with PTSD do. Acute Stress Disorder may precede the development of PTSD. (*DSM-IV 429–430*)

164. Answer is **A**. Often, affected individuals report characteristic symptoms of the disorder in childhood. Children with the disorder are overly conforming, perfectionistic, and unsure of themselves. They may zealously seek approval and require excessive reassurance. In community samples, the lifetime prevalence is 5%, and the one-year prevalence is 3%. The results of studies have been too inconsistent to determine a familial pattern for this disorder. Women make up 55–60% of those affected in clinical settings and two-thirds of the affected population is epidemiological studies. (*DSM-IV 433–434*)

165. Answer is **B**. Both hypothyroidism and hyperthyroidism are associated with this diagnosis. Congestive heart failure and a variety of respiratory conditions may result in this diagnosis, primarily as a result of the lowering of $PO_2$ and the retention of $CO_2$. A $B_{12}$ deficiency may result in anxiety, but thiamine deficiency is most frequently associated with Wernicke's encephalopathy. While knowledge of being HIV positive may induce anxiety in an individual, the virus itself does not cause the anxiety directly. The essential feature of this disorder is the direct production of anxiety symptoms by a medical condition, not the individual's emotional response to a given diagnosis. (*DSM-IV 436–437*)

166. Answer is **D**. This disorder is influenced by cultural factors, and certain prevailing cultural conditions may favor its development. In the United States, the disorder is rarely diagnosed in men, but in other cultures it may be more common in men. Typically, the somatic symptoms of the affected individual do not remit completely, and seldom will a year pass in which the individual does not seek medical attention for unexplained somatic complaints. Some 10% to 20% of female first-degree relatives will have this diagnosis, whereas male relatives of women with the disorder have an increased risk of Antisocial Personality Disorder and Substance-Related Disorders. (*DSM-IV 447*)

167. Answer is **E**. This is a residual category for individuals who present with persistent physical complaints of six months or longer in duration who do not fit the criteria for Somatization Disorder. The most common complaints are chronic fatigue, loss of appetite, and gastrointestinal or genitourinary symptoms. Neurasthenia is described in many parts of the world and is characterized by chronic fatigue and weakness. This diagnosis would be classified as Undifferentiated Somatoform Disorder if symptoms persisted for six months or more. (*DSM-IV 450–451*)

168. Answer is **B**. With chronic pain (six months or longer), Depressive Disorders are more common, and in severe cases suicide may result. With acute pain (less than six months), Anxiety Disorders are more common. DSM-IV requires that psychological factors play a significant role in the onset, maintenance, severity, or exacerbation of the pain, but does not require the absence of demonstrable physical pathology in the patient. Many patients have both demonstrated pathology and the DSM-IV diagnosis of Pain Disorder. The role the pain plays in the life of the individual is key to understanding this diagnosis. (*DSM-IV 458–459*)

169. Answer is **A**. Most commonly, affected individuals have concern about some perceived flaw in their facial characteristics. The concern may be very specific and lead to surgical procedures to correct the "defect." Other body parts, including genitalia, may be perceived as flawed or defective as well. Individuals with this disorder feel that others are taking special notice of their defects and may take extreme measures to prevent others from detecting the "defect." Typically, these individuals are reluctant to talk about the specific perceived defect and may refer to their general ugliness instead. (*DSM-IV 466–467*)

170. Answer is **A**. The disruption of the usually integrated functions of consciousness, memory, identity, and perception is the essence of dissociation. Dissociation itself is not inherently pathological and is a common and expected expression of cultural activities or religious practices in many cultures. The presentation in terms of onset and course may be very variable. A sudden onset may result in dramatic changes, but a more gradual onset may also occur. While some dissociative symptoms may be transient, a chronic course is also possible. These symptoms may be present in a number of disorders, such as stress- or trauma-related disorders. (*DSM-IV 477*)

171. Answer is **D**. This disorder can occur at any age, although in children the diagnosis may be confused with other

diagnoses. Environmental stimuli play a key role in the genesis of this disorder. Traumatic, profoundly disturbing events frequently precede its onset. As with all DSM-IV diagnoses, the affected individual experiences distress or dysfunction as a part of the disorder, and individuals with this disorder are aware of memory gaps, which pose problems for them. (*DSM-IV 478– 479*)

172. Answer is **E**. Unlike the Hypoactive Sexual Desire Disorder the Sexual Aversion Disorder results in feelings of disgust, anxiety, or revulsion in the individual when confronted with a sexual situation. These individuals may avoid all erotic or sensual activity, including kissing and touching. On the other hand, the aversion may be to specific aspects of the sexual experience, such as secretions. Affected individuals may employ many strategies to avoid sexual experience, and marital discord may result. (*DSM-IV 499*)

173. Answer is **C**.    The essential feature of this disorder for women is the inability to maintain the lubrication-swelling response of sexual excitement, and for men it is the inability to attain or maintain an erection to the completion of sexual activity. Disorders of desire are the Hyposexual Desire Disorders. Men with a Sexual Arousal Disorder may have adequate erections in certain situations, and thus are not always impotent. (*DSM-IV 500–501*)

174. Answer is **D**. This disorder is present in men and women and is not caused exclusively by vaginismus or lack of lubrication. The pain may be experienced before, during, and after intercourse. In females, the pain progresses from superficial at intromission to deep during thrusting. (*DSM-IV 511–512*)

# 3

# PSYCHOPHARMACOLOGY

# QUESTIONS

1. Which of the following statements regarding Akathisia is/are true?

   1. Middle-aged women are at increased risk of developing Akathisia.
   2. Akathisia may be misdiagnosed as anxiety or increased psychotic agitation.
   3. Patients with Akathisia may report a sense of anxiety and an inability to relax.
   4. The time course for the development of Akathisia is similar to that of Neuroleptic-Induced Parkinsonism.

2. The anticholinergic drugs are primarily used to treat:

   1. Neuroleptic-Induced Parkinsonism
   2. Neuroleptic-Induced Tremors
   3. Neuroleptic-Induced Acute Dystonia
   4. Lithium-Induced Tremors

3. Which of the following statements regarding the use of physostigmine in the management of anticholinergic intoxication is/are true?

   1. Treatment with physostigmine requires the presence of emergency cardiac monitoring and life support services.
   2. Physostigmine is contraindicated in patients with a history of asthma or cardiac problems.
   3. Physostigmine use should be reserved to confirm a diagnosis of anticholinergic delirium or the treat the most serious symptoms of anticholinergic intoxication.
   4. Physostigmine may be given intravenously (IV) or intramuscularly (IM) with equal effectiveness.

4. Which of the following statements is/are true?

   1. Both benzodiazepine agonists and antagonists bind to the gamma-aminobutyric acid type A (GABA$_A$) receptor complex.
   2. The GABA receptor is G-protein mediated.
   3. Nonbenzodiazepine agonists may be safer and less subject to abuse by patients.
   4. Flumazenil is a potent GABA agonist.

5. Which of the following statements about the metabolism of benzodiazepines is/are true?

   1. Chlordiazepoxide is metabolized to diazepam to desmethyldiazepam to oxazepam to glucuronide.
   2. As a result of the slow metabolism of desmethyldiazepam, all 2-keto benzodiazepines are the longest acting members of this drug group.
   3. Since the attainment of steady–state plasma levels may take up to two weeks, symptoms and signs of toxicity may be manifest 7–10 days after the initiation of treatment at therapeutic doses.
   4. The 3-hydroxy benzodiazepines are directly metabolized by glucuronidation and have no active metabolites.

6. Which of the following statements is/are true?

   1. The omega$_2$ subunit of the GABA$_A$ mediates sleep.
   2. The binding of benzodiazepines to the GABA$_A$ receptors decreases its affinity for gamma-aminobutyric acid.
   3. Binding of benzodiazepine to GABA receptors causes calcium to be actively pumped out of neurons.
   4. Binding of benzodiazepine to GABA receptors causes a flow of chloride ions into the cell via an ionophore.

7. Regarding the adverse effects of the benzodiazepines, which of the following statements is/are true?

   1. The most common side effect of the benzodiazepines is drowsiness, occurring in about 10% of patients.
   2. While ataxia and dizziness are relatively uncommon with benzodiazepine use, falls resulting from these side effects can have serious consequences, especially in the elderly.
   3. Rarely, a paradoxical aggressive reaction may occur in some patients following the ingestion of benzodiazepines, especially in brain-damaged people.
   4. High-potency benzodiazepines can result in antegrade amnesia.

8. Regarding benzodiazepine withdrawal, which of the following statements is/are true?

   1. Abrupt discontinuation of diazepam results in severe and immediate withdrawal.
   2. The fewer the active metabolites a particular benzodiazepine has, the less is the risk of severe and immediate withdrawal symptoms.
   3. Withdrawal symptoms occur only in patients who abuse or take excessive doses of benzodiazepines.
   4. Appearance of withdrawal symptoms may be delayed for up to two weeks when patients stop taking the 2-keto benzodiazepines.

9. Which are correct statements about benzodiazepines and drug interactions?

1. Antacids decrease the absorption of benzodiazepines.
2. Tricyclics taken with benzodiazepines increase depression of the central nervous system (CNS).
3. Cimetidine taken with 2-keto benzodiazepines may increase their blood levels, but it has little effect on lorazepam or oxazepam.
4. Carbamazepine taken with benzodiazepines will increase benzodiazepine blood levels.

10. Which of the following statements concerning buspirone is/are true?

1. Buspirone's effects as an anxiolytic are attributable to its effect on the GABA-associated chloride ion channel.
2. Buspirone decreases the firing rates of serotonergic neurons in the median raphe nucleus and reduces the release of serotonin from the hippocampus.
3. Because of its activity on the GABA receptor, buspirone can be useful in the treatment of withdrawal from benzodiazepines.
4. Studies indicate that buspirone is as effective as benzodiazepines in patients who have not been previously treated with benzodiazepines.

11. Carbamazepine:

1. Is structurally similar to imipramine.
2. Tends to have a shorter half-life with long-term administration due to the induction of hepatic enzymes.
3. Is especially effective in the treatment of temporal lobe epilepsy and trigeminal neuralgia.
4. Has a 10-, 11-epoxide metabolite that is an effective anticonvulsant.

12. Regarding the clinical applications of carbamazepine, which of the following statements is/are correct?

1. Schizophrenic persons with more negative symptoms than positive symptoms may be more likely to respond to carbamazepine.
2. Carbamazepine is an effective antimanic agent in 50–70% of patients and may be with especially useful lithium nonresponders or those with Rapid-Cycling Bipolar Disorder.
3. The positive response rate of depressed patients to carbamazepine is equal to that of standard antidepressants.
4. Carbamazepine may be useful in the management of impulsive and aggressive behavior in nonpsychotic patients.

13. Clozapine differs from traditional antipsychotics in that:

1. It has significantly fewer Parkinsonian-like side effects.
2. It has a much greater affinity for dopamine type 4 receptors.
3. In animal models, it has a more pronounced effect on mesolimbic dopaminergic neurons than on nigrostriatal dopaminergic neurons.
4. It has pronounced serotoninergic effects.

14. Correct statements about the adverse effects of clozapine treatment and the treatment of these unwanted effects are:

1. Sialorrhea, usually worse at night, can be successfully treated with anticholinergic agents.
2. Seizures resulting from clozapine treatment are best remedied by carbamazepine.
3. Mild fevers associated with clozapine can be effectively treated with clonidine patches.
4. Tachycardia secondary to clozapine can be successfully treated with peripherally acting beta-adrenergic antagonists, such as atenolol.

15. Factors that influence the selection of a particular medication include which of the following?

1. Family history of a positive response to a particular medication
2. Patient's history of drug response (compliance, therapeutic response, adverse effects)
3. Target symptoms
4. The treating psychiatrist's usual practice

16. When assessing a therapeutic failure with a medication, which of the following steps should be considered?

1. The diagnosis should be reviewed to determine its accuracy.
2. The dosage and length of time of administration should be carefully reviewed and documented.
3. The potential for interaction with another drug(s) should be assessed.
4. Blood levels should be determined in all medications.

17. Which of the following statements are true regarding the effects of aging on the pharmacokinetics of medication?

1. Total body weight tends to decrease as a result of decreased total body fat.
2. Total body water and plasma albumin decrease with age.
3. Receptor sensitivity decreases with age.
4. Hepatic metabolism of medication tends to decrease with age.

18. Correct statements regarding drug-induced extrapyramidal reactions include:

1. Ninety percent of dystonic reactions will occur within the first week of treatment.
2. Parkinsonism will most likely occur in the second year of treatment.
3. Ninety percent of Akathisia will occur within the first three months of treatment.
4. Young females are most likely to develop dystonic reactions.

19. Which of the following general statements about antipsychotic medications is/are true?

1. Once a patient is stabilized, the antipsychotic medication can be given in a single daily dose.
2. Most antipsychotics are incompletely absorbed after oral administration, although liquid forms are more effectively absorbed than other forms.
3. Intramuscular administration usually results in a more rapid and reliable attainment of therapeutic plasma concentration than does oral administration.
4. The depot formulations of haloperidol and fluphenazine may require up to six months to reach steady-state plasma levels.

20. Which of the following statements is/are true?

    1. The potency of antipsychotic drugs is most closely related to the affinity of these drugs for the $D_2$ receptors.
    2. The dopamine receptor blockage occurs immediately, although the full antipsychotic activity may take weeks to develop.
    3. Most of the neurological and endocrine problems associated with antipsychotic medications can be explained by the blockage of dopamine receptors.
    4. Low pretreatment plasma levels of homovanillic acid may predict for a positive response to antipsychotic medications.

21. Which of the following statements regarding the cardiac effects of antipsychotic medications is/are true?

    1. Chlorpromazine causes prolongation of QT and PR intervals, blunting of T waves, and depression of the ST segment.
    2. Thioridazine may be associated with malignant arrhythmias, such as torsade des pointes.
    3. If QT intervals exceed 0.44 ms, there may be an increased risk of sudden death.
    4. Low-potency antipsychotics are more cardiotoxic than are high-potency antipsychotics.

22. Blockade of the dopamine receptors in the tuberoinfundibular tract results in which of the following?

    1. Breast enlargement
    2. Galactorrhea
    3. Impotence in men
    4. Amenorrhea and inhibited orgasm in women

23. Which of the following statements about neuroleptic-induced parkinsonism is/are true?

    1. Perioral tremors, like other tremors associated with this problem, typically occur late in the course of treatment.
    2. The anticholinergic agents diphenhydramine and amantadine are equally effective in the treatment of this problem.
    3. Neuroleptic-induced parkinsonism usually begins to become apparent after 90 days of treatment.

    4. The differential diagnosis for this clinical problem should include idiopathic parkinsonism, other organic causes of parkinsonism, and depression.

24. Which of the following statements about tardive dyskinesia is/are true?

    1. Perioral movements are the most common.
    2. The dyskinetic movements disappear with sleep and worsen with stress.
    3. Finger movements and hard clenching are common.
    4. About 10–20% of patients treated with antipsychotic mediations for a year will have tardive dyskensia.

25. Which of the following statements about the Neuroleptic Malignant Syndrome (NMS) is/are correct?

    1. The mortality rate may be as high as 30% in patients who develop NMS on depot antipsychotic agents.
    2. Symptoms of NMS typically evolve over 24 to 72 hours, with men more affected more frequently than women.
    3. Autonomic symptoms included hyperpyrexia and increased pulse and blood pressure.
    4. Laboratory findings associated with NMS include leukopenia, elevated creatinine phosphokinase, and elevated myoglobinuria.

26. Which of the following statements about drug interactions and antipsychotics is true?

    1. Antacids taken within two hours of antipsychotic administration can reduce their absorption.
    2. Phenothiazines, especially thioridazine, may decrease the metabolism of diphenylhydantoin.
    3. Coadministration of propranolol with antipsychotics increases the blood levels of both mediations.
    4. Cigarette smoking may decrease the plasma levels of antipsychotics drugs.

27. Factors that influence the dose of an antipsychotic include which of the following?

    1. The therapeutic index for a given antipsychotic is favorable.
    2. The fact that tolerance to side effects develops, but does not develop to the antipsychotic effects
    3. Levels of agitation and violence in patient's presentation
    4. Care giver's desire to achieve rapid results

28. Which of the following statements regarding lithium is/are true?

    1. Lithium reaches peak plasma concentration one to one-and-one-half-hours after ingestion.
    2. Lithium does not cross the blood–brain barrier rapidly.
    3. Lithium is absorbed by the proximal tubules of the kidneys.
    4. Lithium is excreted in breast milk.

29. Which of the following statements concerning lithium's use in special populations is/are true?

1. Adolescents treated with lithium may find the weight gain and acne sometimes associated with lithium especially troubling.
2. Use of lithium during pregnancy may result in Ebstein's anomaly, a malformation of the tricuspid valve.
3. Lithium use in the elderly is safe, however, doses should be changed more slowly than they are for younger patients.
4. If lithium is administered during pregnancy, the lowest possible dose should be used and lithium levels should be closely monitored.

30. Which of the following statements concerning the enzyme monamine oxidase (MAO) is/are true?

   1. Monoamine oxidase is primarily an extracellular enzyme, highly localized in the sympathetic nervous system.
   2. Dietary tyramine is deactivated by MAO in the central nervous system.
   3. Measurement of MAO activity in platelets accurately reflects the degree of MAO inhibition achieved by medication in the central nervous system.
   4. MAO-A is relatively specific for serotonin and norepinephrine, MAO-B is relatively specific for phenylethylamine, and both are involved in the metabolism of dopamine.

31. Which of following statements regarding fluoxetine is/are true?

   1. Norflouxetine, the primary metabolite of fluoxetine, is active in blocking the reuptake of fluoxetine.
   2. Activation and gastrointestinal distress are the two most common side effects of fluoxetine.
   3. Sexual dysfunction occurs in at least 5% of all patients treated with fluoxetine.
   4. Fluoxetine taken during pregnancy does not appear to be associated with fetal abnormalities.

32. Which of the following statements is/are true of tacrine?

   1. The plasma concentration of alanine aminotransferase is the most sensitive indicator of the hepatic effects of tacrine.
   2. The absorption of tacrine is enhanced by taking it with food.
   3. Research indicates that 70% of all patients treated with tacrine will tolerate it over the long term.
   4. The half-life of tacrine is 8–12 hours.

33. Which of the following statements regarding nefazodone is/are true?

   1. The side-effect profile of nefazodone is similar to that of trazodone.
   2. Nefazodone has no active metabolites.
   3. Nefazodone has enduring effects on both norepinephrine and serotonin when patients are maintained on this medication long term.

   4. The primary pharmacodynamic effects of nefazodone are antagonism of the serotonin type 2 receptor and weak inhibitor of serotonin reuptake.

34. Which of the following clinical situations might respond to tricyclic antidepressants?

   1. Panic Disorder with Agoraphobia
   2. Generalized Anxiety Disorder
   3. Chronic Pain Disorders
   4. Obesity management

35. Which of the following statements regarding the termination of tricyclic medications is/are true?

   1. Premature cessation of tricyclic treatment may result in a reemergence of symptoms.
   2. Abrupt cessation may result in a cholinergic rebound syndrome.
   3. Tricyclic and tetracyclic drugs are free of risk for physiological addiction.
   4. The average length of time for tapering tricyclic drugs is two weeks.

36. Which of the following statements is/are true regarding valproate and its interaction with other drugs?

   1. Valproate coadministered with antipsychotics will result in a reduced number of extrapyramidal side effects and a reduced need for antiparkinsonian drugs.
   2. Plasma concentrations of diazepam and phenobarbital will be reduced when coadministered with valproate.
   3. Coadministration with carbamazepine will result in increased plasma concentrations of valproate.
   4. Coadministration with lithium will often exacerbate drug-induced tremors.

37. Which of the following pretreatment evaluations should be done on a patient being considered for electroconvulsive therapy (ECT)?

   1. Blood chemistries, chest X-ray, and an electrocardiogram (ECG)
   2. Spine X-rays, which are required for all patients
   3. Dental examination
   4. Computerized tomography or magnetic resonance imaging of the head

38. Regarding the electrode placement in ECT, which of the following statements is/are true?

   1. Bilateral placement usually results in a more rapid therapeutic response.
   2. Unilateral placement on the nondominant hemisphere may help to reduce the postictal confusion.
   3. Treatment is usually initiated with a unilateral placement.
   4. Indications for bilateral placement include severe depression, mania, catatonic stupor, and treatment-resistant Schizophrenia.

39. Which of the following statements is/are true?

1. For a seizure to be effective in the course of ECT, it must last at least 25 seconds.
2. ECT frequently precipitates a seizure disorder in patients.
3. If a particular stimulus fails to produce a seizure, up to four attempts may be made during that course of treatment.
4. A prolonged seizure is one that lasts longer than 60 seconds.

40. Which of the following statements is/are true?

1. ECT death is usually attributable to cardiovascular causes in patients who already have a compromised cardiac status.
2. Memory impairment is most often reported by patients who experience little improvement from ECT.
3. Most patients return to baseline memory function within six months.
4. The mortality rate for ECT exceeds that for tricyclic antidepressants.

**DIRECTIONS: For questions 41 through 103 select the single best answer.**

41. All of the following statements regarding the interaction of lithium with other drugs are true **EXCEPT**:

a. Thiazide diuretics increase lithium levels
b. Aspirin reduces lithium levels
c. Nonsteroidal anti-inflammatory drugs decrease lithium clearance, and thus increase lithium levels
d. Angiotensin-converting enzyme inhibitors cause lithium concentrations to increase
e. Carbonic anhydrase inhibitors and xanthines (caffeine) reduce lithium levels

42. All of the following statements concerning the initiation of lithium treatment are true **EXCEPT**:

a. Laboratory evaluations of renal, thyroid, and hematopoietic systems and pregnancy status should be performed before starting lithium treatment.
b. For most adults, the usual starting dose is 300 mg, three times a day.
c. Maintenance lithium levels should be 0.6–1.2 Eq/L
d. Lithium levels are best determined by drawing blood 18 hours after the last dose.
e. Single daily dosing with lithium is not considered to current standard practice.

43. All of the following statements regarding medication-induced tremors are true **EXCEPT**:

a. A variety of psychiatric medications—neuroleptic, lithium, and antidepressants—can produce tremors.
b. The tremors usually decrease during periods of relaxation and worsen when the patient is angry or tense.
c. Medications should be reduced to the lowest possible dosage and be taken at bedtime to minimize daytime tremors.

d. Caffeine may reduce daytime tremors.
e. ß-adrenergic receptor antagonists may reduce tremors.

44. Correct statements regarding the use of propranolol in patients with psychiatric conditions include all of the following **EXCEPT**:

a. Propranolol is an effective treatment for Acute Akathisia, Acute Dystonia and parkinsonism.
b. Some studies indicate that propranolol may be helpful in controlling aggression and violent behavior in certain patients.
c. Propranolol may be a useful adjuvant, but not the sole treatment, in the management of Alcohol Withdrawal syndrome.
d. Use of propranolol should be avoid in patients with diabetes mellitus because the drug will antagonize the normal physiological response to hypoglycemia.
e. The performance type of Social Phobia may respond especially well to propranolol treatment.

45. Current therapeutic uses for the use of barbiturates in psychiatric practice include all of the following **EXCEPT**:

a. Amobarbital can be use intramuscularly (IM) to control agitation in emergency situations.
b. Phenobarbital is the barbiturate of choice when detoxifying a patient from barbiturate dependence.
c. Barbiturates are primarily drugs for the management of insomnia.
d. The Phenobarbital Challenge Test is a safe and effective maneuver to asses a patient's tolerance to barbiturates.
e. Amobarbital can be used for diagnostic interviews.

46. All of the following statements about benzodiazepine and barbiturates are true **EXCEPT**:

a. Barbiturates are schedule II drugs and benzodiazepines are schedule IV drugs by Drug Enforcement Agency classification.
b. Both have a low therapeutic index.
c. Both have additive and abuse potential.
d. Both have potential teratogenic effects.
e. Both have seizure activity as a potential problem in acute withdrawal.

47. All of the following statements regarding benzodiazepines are true **EXCEPT**:

a. All benzodiazepines are completely absorbed unchanged from the gastrointestinal tract.
b. The benodiazepines having the quickest absorption, attainment of peak levels, and onset of action are diazepam, lorazepam, alprazolam, triazolam, and estazolam.
c. Plasma levels of benzodiazepines are biphasic: a peak at initial absorption and a peak later, secondary to enterohepatic circulation.
d. Only lorazepam is reliably absorbed from IM injection sites.

e. Benzodiazepines are highly lipid soluble, a characteristic that may vary fivefold among members of this drug class.

48. Therapeutic actions of benzodiazepines include all of the following **EXCEPT**:

a. Anticonvulsant activity
b. Skeletal muscle relaxation
c. Insomnia
d. Anxiety reduction
e. Treatment of Acute Dystonia

49. Symptoms that are more likely to represent true benzodiazepine withdrawal rather than a return or exacerbation of the original Anxiety Disorder include all of the following **EXCEPT**:

a. Nausea
b. Headache
c. Depersonalization
d. Clinical depression
e. Altered perception

50. All of the following statements regarding the discontinuation of benzodiazepine treatment are true **EXCEPT**:

a. After long-term use of benzodiazepines, 90% of patients will experience some form of withdrawal, even if the drug is tapered slowly.
b. The higher the dose and the shorter the half half-life, the more sever will be the withdrawal.
c. The higher the dose and the longer the half-life, the more severe will be the withdrawal.
d. The drug should not be reduced by more than 25% per week in order to minimize withdrawal and to prevent rebound anxiety.
e. Concurrent use of carbamazepine and supportive psychotherapy may be helpful during the tapering of the medication.

51. Which of the following statements about zolpidem is true?

a. Zolpidem is chemically related to the benodiazepines.
b. Zolpidem has greater affinity for $BZ_2$ receptors than for $BZ_1$ receptors.
c. Zolpidem's strong affinity for peripheral benzodiazepine receptors accounts of its potent muscle relaxant properties.
d. Zolpidem has no active metabolites.
e. Tolerance and dependence are common problems with this drug.

52. All of the following statements about carbamazepine are true **EXCEPT**:

a. Carbamazepine is associated with a benign decrease in the white blood cell (WBC) count, with values always remaining above 3,000.
b. The WBC count decrease is thought to be caused by the inhibition of colony-stimulating factor, an effect that can be reversed by lithium.

c. Carbamazepine has an apparent vasopressin-like effect that can produce hypernatremia, especially in the elderly.
d. Carbamazepine may produce an increase in urinary free cortisol.
e. Carbamazepine decreases atrioventricular (A-V) conduction, and thus should not be used in patients with A-V heart blocks.

53. All of following statements regarding the adverse effects of carbamazepine are true **EXCEPT**:

a. There does not appear to be a correlation between the degree of benign WBC suppression and the emergence of life-threatening blood dyscrasias.
b. The development of a hypersensitivity hepatitis, with increases in liver enzymes and cholestasis, is an absolute contraindication to reintroducing carbamazepine to a patient so affected.
c. The most common adverse effects of carbamazepine are drowsiness, confusion, and ataxia.
d. Elderly patients and patients with cognitive disorders are at increased risk for central nervous system CNS carbamazepine.
e. Minor cranial–facial abnormalities and spina bifida may be associated with maternal use of carbamazepine during pregnancy.

54. All of the following statements concerning carbamazepine administration are true **EXCEPT**:

a. Prior to initiating treatment, any preexisting hematological, hepatic, and cardiac conditions must be investigated thoroughly.
b. The Food and Drug Administration (FDA) suggests complete blood counts (CBC) every two weeks for the first two months of treatment and quarterly thereafter.
c. The usual starting dose of carbamazepine is 200 mg twice a day, increased by 200 mg increments every two to four days.
d. When discontinuing carbamazepine, a tapered dosage is not necessary.
e. The average therapeutic total daily dose of carbamazepine is 1,000 mg.

55. When using clozapine, the patient may experience all of the following adverse effects **EXCEPT**:

a. Increased risk of seizures
b. Acute Dystonia
c. Drowsiness
d. Agranulocytosis in 1–2% of patients
e. Trachycardia due to vagal inhibition

56. Which of the following statements about tricyclic antidepressants (TCAs) is true?

a. Amitriptyline is a secondary amine.
b. Side effects of TCAs are more pronounced with secondary amines.
c. TCAs inhibit the reuptake of norepinephrine within hours of the first dose.

d. TCAs up/regulate ß-adrenergic receptors in the brain.

e. TCAs stimulate an increased production of CNS monoamines.

57. Which of the following statements is true?

a. The tertiary amines more potentially inhibit the reuptake of serotonin than does norepinephrine.

b. Orthostatic hypotension may result from intense anticholinergic activity of the tertiary amines.

c. Antihistaminic effects may result in dry mouth and urinary retention.

d. Tricyclics exert a digitalis-like effect on cardiac function.

e. Depression of CNS respiratory centers is a major complication of a tricyclic overdose.

58. Which of the following statements about the enzyme monamine oxidase (MAO) is true?

a. MAO is the predominant means of removal of monoamines from the synaptic cleft.

b. MAO is exclusively extracellular.

c. MAO degrades norepinephrine and dopamine, but not serotonin.

d. MAO exists in a mixture of two subtypes—A and B.

e. MAO-B deaminates norepinephrine.

59. Which of the following antidepressants poses the highest risk of seizure?

a. Trazodone

b. Amitriptyline

c. Fluoxetine

d. Phenelzine

e. Bupropion

60. All of the following statements regarding are true EXCEPT:

a. Bupropion bears some structural similarity to dopamine.

b. Bupropion does not affect neurotransmitter systems other than dopaminergic systems.

c. Bupropion weakly inhibits the dopamine reuptake pump.

d. Like amphetamine, bupropion is taken up by the dopamine reuptake pump and is stored in presynaptic vesicles.

e. Bupropion lacks the addictive qualities of amphetamine.

61. Nausea is a common side effect of all of the following antidepressants EXCEPT:

a. Venlafaxine

b. Bupropion

c. Setraline

d. Paroxetine

e. Fluoxetine

62. All of the following statements about AIDS Dementia Due to HIV Disease are true EXCEPT:

a. Patients may experience significant problems with balance, especially with rapid head turns.

b. Aphasia may be a prominent feature of the clinical presentation.

c. Typically, these patients are withdrawn and amotivational late in the course of the illness.

d. Dementia typically develops in the late stages of AIDS, but may rarely occur much earlier in the course of the illness.

e. The classic triad of AIDS dementia is problems with cognitive, behavior, and motor function.

63. The most common psychiatric problem among HIV-infected patients is:

a. Depression

b. Dementia

c. Substance abuse

d. Sexual dysfunction

e. Adjustment Disorder

64. All of the following influence a medication's distribution to the brain following an oral dose. Which would be least predictive of the ultimate delivery to the neural receptor?

a. Blood–brain barrier

b. Brain's regional blood flow

c. Drug's affinity for receptors

d. Amount of oral dose

e. Net gastrointestinal (GI) absorption of drug

65. Potential adverse effects caused by blockade of muscarinic acetylcholine receptors include all of the following EXCEPT:

a. Blurred vision

b. Decreased sweating

c. Urinary retention

d. Retrograde ejaculation

e. Orthostatic hypotension

66. The usual pattern of symptoms following a tricyclic overdose is:

a. Initially, a profound CNS depression with areflexia and decorticate posturing, followed by hyperarousal, and then cardiovascular collapse.

b. Respiratory depression with skeletal muscle fasciculation and hypothermia followed by seizures and coma.

c. Initial CNS stimulation with confusion, agitation, and hallucinations, followed by CNS depression with respiratory depression and cardiac conduction problems.

d. Severe GI upset secondary to hypermotility followed by slow onset of coma.

e. Tachyarhythmia with syncope and confusion followed by bradyarrhythmia with concomitant coma.

67. If the amount of tricyclic antidepressant ingested in an overdose is unknown, the best indicator of the severity of the overdose may be:

a. Degree of hyperreflexia
b. Degree of QRS prolongation on the electrocardiogram (ECG)
c. Degree of respiratory depression as measured by arterial blood gases
d. Degree of positive response to physostigmine infusion
e. Degree of decrease in bowel sounds

68. Risk factors for the development of Neuroleptic-Induced Tardive Dyskinesia include all of the following **EXCEPT**:

a. Long-term treatment with neuroleptics
b. Presence of a Mood Disorder
c. Presence of a cognitive disorder
d. Male sex
e. Increasing age

69. Which of the following statements about lithium is/are true?

a. Lithium is bound to plasma proteins.
b. Lithium is distributed nonuniformly throughout total body water.
c. Lithium rapidly crosses the blood–brain barrier after ingestion.
d. Lithium is almost entirely excreted by the kidneys.

70. All of the following statements concerning lithium's effects on specific organ systems are true **EXCEPT**:

a. Lithium enhances the release of thyroid hormone from the thyroid and can result in goiter.
b. Lithium may impair sinus mode function, which can result in heart block.
c. Lithium may reduce the kidney's ability to concentrate urine, resulting in nephrogenic diabetes insipidus.
d. Lithium causes a leukocytosis as a result of an increase colony maturation factor secretion.
e. Thyroid problems as a result of lithium administration occur more frequently in women than in men.

71. All of the following factors are indictors for maintaining a patient on lithium after the person's first manic episode **EXCEPT**:

a. The patient has a family history of Bipolar I Disorder.
b. There are no precipitating factors for the first episode.
c. The patient is a high suicide risk.
d. The patient is 30 years of age or older.
e. The patient is female.

72. All of the following statements concerning lithium-induced tremor are true **EXCEPT**:

a. Tremor is most prominent in the fingers.
b. The tremor is unrelated to the plasma level of lithium.
c. Propranolol may be effective in reducing the tremor in many patients.
d. Less than 10% of lithium-treated patients experience tremors.

73. All of the following statements concerning the renal effects of lithium are true **EXCEPT**:

a. Polyuria seen with lithium is due to the antagonistic effect on antidiuretic hormone at the distal tubules.
b. The problem affects 25–30% of lithium-treated patients.
c. The polyuria may result in dehydration that may require fluid replacement.
d. Treatment of polyuria secondary to lithium administration may be the use of a thiazide diuretic, in which case the lithium dose should be increased to compensate for its greater excretion.
e. The incidence of severe renal complications is now thought to be lower than originally believed.

74. Correct statements regarding drug interactions with clozapine include all of the following **EXCEPT**:

a. CNS depressants, alcohol, or tricyclic drugs coadministered with clozapine may increase the incidence of seizures, sedation, and cardiac effects.
b. Propylthiouracil, sulfonamides, and captopril can be used safely in clozapine-treated patients.
c. Rarely, respiratory depression may result when benzodiazepines are used in clozapine-treated patients.
d. A combination of benzodiazepine and clozapine may result in an increased incidence of orthostasis and syncope.
e. Lithium combined with clozapine may increase the risk of seizure, confusion, and movement disorders.

75. Which of the following statements is true?

a. The initial dosage of clozapine is usually 25 mg per day or 25 mg twice a day.
b. One milligram of clozapine is equivalent to 3 to 5 mg of chlorpromazine.
c. Clozapine should be tapered slowly when it is discontinued to prevent rebound cholinergic symptoms, such as diaporesis, flushing, and diarrhea.
d. The usual therapeutic dose of clozapine is 150–200 mg.

76. All of the following statements about disulfiram are true **EXCEPT**:

a. Disulfiram is almost completely absorbed from the GI tract, is metabolized by the liver, and is excreted in urine.
b. Disulfiram is an aldehyde dehydrogenase inhibitor that interferes with the metabolism of alcohol and produces a marked increase in blood aldehyde levels.
c. Extreme disulfiram–alcohol reactions may result in respiratory depression, myocardial infarction, cardiovascular collapse, convulsions, and death.
d. Disulfiram decreases the blood concentration of diazepam, phenytoin, anticoagulants, and tricyclic drugs.
e. The usual dosage is 500 mg per day for the first one to two weeks and then 250 mg per day, with careful monitoring for compliance and adverse effects.

77. Cardiac effects of antipsychotic drugs include all of the following **EXCEPT**:

    a. Reduction of coronary artery flow
    b. Decreased myocardial contractility
    c. Increased atrial and ventricular conduction times
    d. Increased length of refractory time

78. Potential problems encountered with the antipsychotic medications include all of the following **EXCEPT**:

    a. Dry mouth and constipation
    b. Skin rashes and discoloration
    c. Leukocytosis
    d. Sexual dysfunction
    e. Orthostatic hypotension

79. Regarding the therapeutic responses to antipsychotics, which of the following statements is incorrect?

    a. Antipsychotic medications are thought to be more effective in the treatment of the positive symptoms of Schizophrenia than the negative symptoms.
    b. Antipsychotic medications may contribute to the development of negative symptoms.
    c. Paranoid patients may respond better than nonparanoid patients.
    d. Fifty percent of persons with Schizophrenia relapse on maintenance antipsychotic medications during their first year of treatment.
    e. Patients with Schizophrenia who relapse while on maintenance neuroleptics have less severe symptoms than do those not receiving antipsychotic medications.

80. All of the following statements about the effects of antipsychotics on the hematopoietic system are correct **EXCEPT**:

    a. A transient leukopenia (about 3,500 WBC) may be seen when initiating these medications.
    b. Agranulocytosis occurs most frequently with chlorpromazine and thioridazine, but can be seen with almost all antipsychotics.
    c. Agranulocytosis usually occurs after a year or more of treatment with antipsychotics.
    d. The incidence of agranulocytosis is about five patients per 10,000.
    e. The mortality rate for agranulocytosis caused by antipsychotics may be as high as 30%.

81. Correct statements about the opthalmological effects of antipsychotics include all of the following **EXCEPT**:

    a. Thioridazine is associated with pigmentation of the retina in doses of more than 800 mg per day.
    b. The pigmentation seen with thioridazine is similar to that of retinitis pigmentosa.
    c. The pigmentation slowly reverses once the thioridazine is stopped.
    d. Chlorpromazine is associated with benign granular deposits in the anterior lens and posterior cornea.
    e. Retinal damage is not seen in patients treated with chlorpromazine.

82. All of the following statements concerning Neuroleptic-Induced Parkinsonism are true **EXCEPT**:

    a. Parkinsonian adverse effects occur in about 15% of patients who are treated with antipsychotics.
    b. A positive glabellar tap reflex involves a failure of the orbicularis oculi to accommodate to repeated taps between the eyebrows.
    c. Women and men are equally at risk for this adverse effect.
    d. All antipsychotics can cause this problem, but especially high-potency drugs with low anticholinergic activity.
    e. Blockade of dopaminergic transmission in the nigrostriatal tract is the cause of Neuroleptic-Induced Parkinsonism.

83. All of the following statements about Neuroleptic-Induced Acute Dystonia are true **EXCEPT**:

    a. Dystonic reactions affect about 10% of all patients and usually occur within hours to days after treatment is started.
    b. Unlike in other types of Dystonia, oculogyric crisis may occur late in treatment.
    c. Children are especially likely to evidence opisthotonos, scoliosis, lordosis, and writhing movements.
    d. Dystonia is most common in men under the age of 40.
    e. The mechanism of action is probably dopaminergic hyperactivity in the motor cortex, occurring when CNS levels of antipsychotics fall between doses.

84. All of the following statements regarding Tardive Dyskinesia are true **EXCEPT**:

    a. Tardive Dyskinesia evolves slowly and follows a relentlessly chronic and progressive course.
    b. Tardive Dyskinesia may be caused by dopaminergic receptor supersensitivity in the basal ganglia, resulting from chronic blockade of dopamine receptors by antipsychotic medication.
    c. Prevention of Tardive Dyskinesia is best achieved by using antipsychotics only when indicated and at the lowest possible dose.
    d. Patients receiving antipsychotic medications should have regular standardized evaluations for the presence of movement disorder.
    e. Some 50–90% of mild cases of Tardive Dyskinesia remit spontaneously.

85. Major contraindications to the administration of antipsychotics include all of the following **EXCEPT**:

    a. A high risk of seizures from idiopathic or organic causes
    b. A history of asthma

c. Presence of narrow-angle glaucoma
d. History or presence of Tardive Dyskinesia
e. Presence of severe cardiac disease

86. Correct statements regarding lithium's effects on organ systems include all of following **EXCEPT**:

a. Polyuria secondary to lithium's antagonism of antidiuretic hormone may be present in 25–35% of lithium-treated patients.
b. Gastrointestinal complaints are the most common adverse effects of lithium.
c. The cardiac effects of lithium resemble those of hypokalemia on the ECG.
d. Lithium suppresses the secretion of thyroid-stimulating hormone.
e. Lithium stimulates the production of colony-stimulating factor, resulting in a benign leukocytosis.

87. Correct statements regarding the adverse effects of monoamine oxidase inhibitors (MAOIs) include all of the following **EXCEPT**:

a. Weight gain, edema, and sexual dysfunction as a result of MAOI treatment usually respond to treatment and are not indicative of a need to change to another medication.
b. Hypertensive crises may occur in patients treated with MAOIs as a result of the MAOI itself.
c. MAOIs are frequently associated with hypotension.
d. Phenelzine and isocardoxazid are associated with significant hepatoxicity.
e. Over-the-counter cold and allergy remedies should be avoided.

88. Which of the following statements regarding fluoxetine is true?

a. Fluoxetine cannot be mixed with warfarin.
b. Fluoxetine may require up to two weeks to achieve steady-state concentrations.
c. Fluoxetine can be coadministered with tricyclic medications at low doses.
d. When changing from fluoxetine to an MAOI, one week should elapse between the medications.
e. Fluoxetine cannot be coadministered with sympathomimetics.

89. All of the following statements about sympathomimetics are true **EXCEPT**:

a. The primary action of sympathomimetics is to cause the release of dopamine into the synaptic cleft.
b. Dextroamphetamine and methylphenidate are structurally similar to amphetamine and to catecholamines.
c. Long-term use of sympathomimetics results in tolerance to both the euphoric effects and the sympathomimetic effects.
d. Dextroamphetamine is usually given in a single daily dose.

e. Sympathomimetics can be used in combination with antidepressants.

90. All of the following statements about tacrine are true **EXCEPT**:

a. The primary action of tacrine is the inhibition of acetylcholinesterase.
b. Tacrine must be given three times a day owing to its rapid excretion.
c. Tacrine is used for mildly to moderately demented patients suffering from Dementia of the Alzheimer's Type.
d. Activation of the parasympathetic nervous system may result in nausea, vomiting, and diarrhea.
e. Approximately 5% of patients treated with tacrine have elevated serum glutamic-oxaluacetic transaminase (SGOT) and serum glutamic-pyruvic transaminase (SGPT).

91. All of the following statements regarding trazodone are true **EXCEPT**:

a. Trazodone has moderate anticholinergic activity.
b. The half-life of trazodone is 6–11 hours.
c. Trazodone is a relatively specific inhibitor of serotonin reuptake.
d. The alpha-adrenergic antagonist activity may result in priapism is small percentage of patients.
e. Trazodone can be used as hypnotic.

92. Correct statements regarding the pharmacokinetics of tricyclic antidepressants include all of the following **EXCEPT**:

a. Tricyclic medications are highly protein bound.
b. Absorption of these compounds is complete from the GI tract.
c. Half-lives of tricyclic medications vary widely.
d. Significant first-pass metabolism results is the conversion of many tertiary amines to secondary amines.
e. Many tricyclic drugs are metabolized by the hepatic enzyme $P_{450}IID6$.

93. All of the following statements regarding the pharmacodynamics of tricyclic and tetracyclic drugs are true **EXCEPT**:

a. The reduction of serotonin and norepinephrine reuptake occurs within minutes to hours after an oral dose.
b. These medications block muscarinic acetylcholine and histamine receptors.
c. Long-term administration of these drugs results in the down-regulation of beta-adrenergic receptors and perhaps $5HT_2$ receptors.
d. The down-regulation of beta-adenoreceptors correlates it the time needed to achieve antidepressant effects.
e. Imipramine is the most potent antihistaminic of all the tricyclics.

94. All of the following statements regarding potential adverse effects of tricyclic drugs are true **EXCEPT**:

    a. The sedative effect of tricyclic drugs is due to effects on noradrenergic systems.
    b. Anticholinergic effects are common, but tolerance to these effects will frequently develop.
    c. The most common autonomic nervous system effect is orthostatic hypotension.
    d. Imipramine has a quinidinelike effect on myocardial conduction and may reduce premature ventricular contractions at therapeutic levels.
    e. Weight gain due to blockade of histamine type 2 receptors is common.

95. Correct statements about drug interactions of tricyclic and tetracyclic drugs with other medications include all of the following **EXCEPT**:

    a. Tricyclic and tetracyclic drugs block the neuronal uptake of guanethidine, which is necessary for its action.
    b. Plasma levels of tricyclic drugs are decreased when coadministered with antipsychotics.
    c. Oral contraceptives may decrease tricyclic and tetracyclic plasma levels.
    d. The antihypertensive effects of beta-adrenergic receptor antagonists may be blocked by tricyclic and tetracyclic drugs.
    e. The CNS depressants have additive sedative effects when coadministered with tricyclic or tetracyclic drugs.

96. Which of the following statements regarding valproate is true?

    a. Valproate is chemically related to carbamazepine.
    b. Valproate's favorable action in Bipolar I Disorder is mediated by its suppression of the locus ceruleus.
    c. The most common adverse effect associated with valproate is GI distress in about 25% of patients.
    d. Valproate suppresses the appetite and may aggravate Anorexia Nervosa in depressed patients.
    e. Valproate use during pregnancy is associated with cardiac defects in the fetus.

97. All of the following statements about venlafaxine are true **EXCEPT**:

    a. Venlafaxine may have a slower onset of action than other antidepressants but is as effective.
    b. Venlafaxine has a half-life of five hours, thus requiring multiple doses during the day.
    c. Venlafaxine is a nonselective reuptake inhibitor of norepinephrine, serotonin, and dopamine.
    d. Some patients (3%) experience hypertension on high doses of venlafaxine.
    e. Venlafaxine has at least one active metabolite.

98. In which of the following diagnoses would ECT be a potential treatment choice?

    a. Schizophrenia
    b. Major Depression Disorder
    c. Catatonic Disorder
    d. Bipolar Disorder
    e. Obsessive-Compulsive Disorder

99. All of the following medications should be withdrawn before the initiation of ECT **EXCEPT**:

    a. Tricyclics
    b. Clozapine
    c. Benzodiazepines
    d. Lithium
    e. Theophylline

100. All of the following statements regarding seizure threshold and ECT are true **EXCEPT**:

    a. Seizure thresholds vary little among patients.
    b. During the course of the ECT, the patient's seizure threshold may increase up to 200%.
    c. Seizure thresholds are generally higher in men than in women.
    d. Elderly patients have a higher seizure threshold than do young adults.
    e. A common technique is to start ECT at an electrical stimulus thought to be subthreshold and to increase the stimulus by 100% in unilateral placement and by 50% in bilateral placement.

101. All of the following statements about the number and spacing of ECT treatments are true **EXCEPT**:

    a. The treatments are administered two to three times a week.
    b. The usual course of treatment is six to 12 treatments.
    c. The treatment of Catatonic Disorder usually requires more treatments than does any other condition.
    d. If a patient is not improving after six to 10 sessions, bilateral, high-intensity treatment should be attempted before ECT is abandoned.
    e. The point of maximal improvement is the point at which the patient fails to improve after two consecutive treatments.

102. All of the following statements about the contraindications to ECT are correct **EXCEPT**:

    a. There are no absolute contraindications.
    b. Pregnancy is not a contraindication to ECT, but fetal monitoring is required on all cases, high risk or not.
    c. Patients with a recent myocardial infarction are a high-risk group, although the risk is greatly reduced two weeks after the myocardial infarction.
    d. Patients with hypertension should be stabilized on their medications before ECT is initiated.
    e. Patients with space-occupying lesions are at risk for brain edema and herniation with ECT.

103. All of the following statements are true about phototherapy (light therapy) **EXCEPT**:

a. Exposure to light in the morning is most effective in treating depression.
b. Full-spectrum light, not narrow-spectrum light is effective.
c. Thirty minutes of light exposure is as effective as two hours.
d. The major indication for phototherapy is the Mood Disorder with Seasonal Patterns.
e. The treatment requires light that is 200 times brighter than normal indoor lighting.

# ANSWERS AND EXPLANATIONS

1. Answer is **E**. Middle-aged women have an increased risk for the development of akathisia. Frequently misdiagnosed as anxiety or increased psychotic agitation, patients report feeling tense and anxious. Repetitive movements, such as pacing or rocking, may be observed. Both Neuroleptic-Induced Parkinsonism and akathisia usually develop within the first 90 days of treatment. *(SP 885)*

2. Answer is **A**. Neuroleptic-Induced Parkinsonism, tremors, and acute dystonia are all indications for the use of anticholinergic medications. Lithium-induced tremors respond best to low-dose propranolol *(SP 896)*

3. Answer is **A**. Physostigmine is erratically absorbed from IM injection. Since the potential for severe life-threatening adverse reactions to physostigmine exists, its use is restricted to sites with adequate medical support and is reserved only for diagnosis or treatment of severe symptomatology. Patients with unstable vital signs, asthma, or a history of cardiac abnormalities should not receive physostigmine. *(SP 898)*

4. Answer is **B**. The GABA receptor has sites for the binding of both benzodiazepine agonists and antagonists. The new nonbenzodiazepine agonists, such as zolpidem, may be safer and have less abuse potential than the currently available benzodiazepines. The GABA receptor complex is a chloride ion ionophore type of receptor and is not G-protein mediated. Flumazenil is a potent GABA receptor antagonist and is used to reverse the action of benzodiazepines, usually in overdose situations. *(SP 906)*

5. Answer is **E**. All of these statements are true. The metabolic pathway for chlordiazepoxide is well known and results in a number of active metabolites. Desmethydiazepam is the rate-limiting step and its slow metabolism results in long half-lives of the 2-keto benzodiazepines and the slow attainment of steady-state equilibrium. Thus a dose initially thought to be therapeutic may produce adverse or toxic effects as long as 7–10 days after initiation of treatment. The hydroxy-benodiazepines are directly metabolized via glucuronidation, giving them short half-lives and no active metabolites. *(SP 907)*

6. Answer is **D**. GABA receptors are chloride ionophores. When benzodiazepines bind to GABA, the affinity for gamma-aminobutyric acid is increased, thus causing the ion channel to open. Calcium flux across neuronal membranes is most likely mediated by NMDA receptors, not the GABA system. *(SP 908)*

7. Answer is **E**. Although drowsiness is the most common adverse effect from the use of benzodiazepines, ataxia and dizziness may occur and result in falls, with subsequent fractures. Some patients do respond paradoxically to these drugs, displaying agitation or aggression. This is especially true of patients with brain injury. Patients taking benzodiazepines may conduct themselves normally, but may be alarmed that they have no memory for events, conversations, etc. This amnestic effect has been exploited by anesthesiology, and benzodiazepines have long been used as amnestic adjuvants. *(SP 911)*

8. Answer is **D**. The 2-keto benzodiazepines have multiple active metabolites that delay the onset of withdrawal symptoms. Diazepam is a 2-keto benzodiazepine. The fewer the active metabolites, the greater is the risk of a withdrawal symptoms. Withdrawal symptoms may occur in any patient, including those who are compliant with the psychiatrist's instructions. A careful taper of these medications is always required. *(SP 911)*

9. Answer is **A**. Antacids and food may decrease the absorption from the gut. Tricyclic antidepressants, antihistamines, and alcohol all increase the CNS depressant effect of benzodiazepines. The 2-keto benzodiazepines have a complex metabolism with many active metabolites produced. Cimetidine may slow this process, resulting in an increase in active metabolites and subsequent toxicity. Lorazepam and oxazepam are directly glucuronidated and produce no active metabolites. Carbamazepines, and possibly other anticonvulsants, decrease the blood level of benzodiazepines by the induction of hepatic enzymes when the two are taken concurrently. *(SP 912)*

10. Answer is **C**. Buspirone does decrease serotonergic neuronal firing in the median raphe nucleus and reduce the release of serotonin in the hippocampus. Although many clinicians remain unconvinced of buspirones efficacy, studies indicate that in benzodiazepine-naive patients, buspirone is as effective as the benzodiazepines for generalized anxiety disorder. Buspirone's effects are due to its partial agonist activity on the serotonin type $1_A$ receptors, not on the GABA receptor system. This lack of activity on the GABA system makes buspirone unsuitable for use in the treatment of withdrawal from benzodiazepines, alcohol, or sedative hypnotics. *(SP 921–922)*

11. Answer is **E**. Carbamazepine has a chemical structure similar to that of imipramine. It is erratically absorbed from the gastrointestinal tract and has a wide range of half-lives at the initiation of treatment. Both trigeminal neuralgia and temporal lobe epilepsy respond well to carbamazepine, and the 10-, 11-epoxide metabolite is active as an anticonvulsant. *(SP 925)*

12. Answer is **C**. More positive symptoms in persons with Schizophrenia tend to predict for a positive response to carbamazepine. Carbamazepine is an effective antimanic medication, with 50–70% of patients responding positively, and may be especially helpful in the treatment of lithium nonresponders and those with Rapid Cycling Bipolar Disorders. Up to a third of depressed patients may respond to carbamazepine treatment, a rate far lower than the rate for standard antidepressants. Aggressive, impulsive behavior in nonpsychotic patients may be successfully treated with this drug. *(SP 926)*

13. Answer is **E**. One of the distinct advantages of clozapine is its relative absence of parkinsonian-like effects. This may be due to its greater specificity in the dopaninergic system. It has a much higher affinity for $D_4$ receptors than for $D_2$ receptors and affects mesolimbic structures more than it does nigrostriatal neuons. Additionally, clozapine's potent serotoninergic activity may play an important role in its success in the treatment of the negative symptoms of Schizophrenia. *(SP 932–933)*

14. Answer is **D**. The vagal inhibitory effects of clozapine can be successfully treated with peripherally acting beta-adrenergic antagonists. Unfortunately, such treatment may aggravate the hypotensive effects of clozapine, and thus a careful investigation of the tachycardia is warranted before beginning treatment. Additional anticholinergic agents should be avoided due to the potent anticholinergic activity of clozapine. Some reports indicate that clonidine patches or low-dose amitriptyline may be helpful for sialorrhea. Carbamazepine should not be use in clozapine-treated patients because of its association with agranulocytosis. Phenobarbital can be useful in the management of these seizures. Any reported fevers with clozapine use must be thoroughly evaluated. Agranulocytosis and neuroleptic malignant syndrome must be included in the differential diagnosis and the medication withheld while the evaluation in under way. *(SP 934–935)*

15. Answer is **E**. All of these factors play a role in the selection of a particular medication for a patient. Often a family's response to particular agent will predict for others in the family. The particular agent will predict for others in the family. The patient's approach to medication in terms of willingness to take the medication, ability to tolerate adverse effects, and so on, would play a central role in drug selection. Clearly defined target symptoms, combined with a knowledge of the psychopharmacology of particular medication, produce rational choices. The psychiatrist's knowledge, experience, and training play an important role in the approach to treatment with medication. *(SP 868)*

16. Answer is **A**. Accurate diagnosis is essential for effective treatment planning. Many patients experience a failure because the dose was too low and the medication was taken for too short a time. Drug–drug interactions are quite common with both prescription and over-the-counter medications. A careful investigation of all medications is required. Blood levels are useful with some medications but not universally so. Patients may have therapeutic blood levels but fail to achieve therapeutic results. Peripheral blood levels also may not reflect the concentration in the central nervous system. The patient's clinical response ultimately is more important than any laboratory value. *(SP 869)*

17. Answer is **C**. Total body water and albumin decrease with age, resulting in a decreased volume of distribution for water-soluble drugs and more unbound (free) drug in the plasma. Hepatic enzyme activity generally decreases with age, resulting in prolonged half-lives of drugs. Although, the total body weight tends to decrease with age, this is due to a loss of lean body mass. Total body fat tends to increase. Receptor sensitivity affinity may increase with age, resulting in a greater sensitivity to medication. *(SP 871–872)*

18. Answer is **B**. Most dystonic reactions occur promptly after the initiation of treatment, usually within the first days. Akathisia is a very common side effect, and most of it will be reported in the first three months of treatment. Parkinsonism also occurs in the first three months of treatment. Young males are at highest risk for the development of dystonic reactions. *(SP 882)*

19. Answer is **E**. After a period of initial stabilization, antipsychotics may be given in single daily doses. By taking the medication at bedtime, adverse effects may be reduced. Also, single daily doses improve compliance. Oral liquid preparations and intramuscular administration are superior to oral administration of pills in the attainment of therapeutic blood levels rapidly and reliably. The depot formulations of haloperidol and fluphenazine are esters of the parent compound mixed with sesame seed oil. The rate of entry into the body is determined by rate of diffusion of the esterified compound into the body from the oil. Then the esterified drug is rapidly hydrolyzed, releasing active drug. This produces a very long half-life, and steady state may take up to six months to achieve. Oral administration of medication may have to be continued for the first month following the depot injection. *(SP 944)*

20. Answer is **A**. The $D_2$ receptor seems to play a central role in the mediation of psychosis and its treatment. The affinity for the antipsychotic medication for this receptor and its resultant blockage is most closely correlated with the drug's potential for reducing psychotic symptomatology. Unfortunately, many of the unwanted effects of antipsychotics (e.g., movement disorders, prolactin increases)

may also be linked to the blockage of this receptor. This blockade occurs within minutes to hours after ingestion, but the therapeutic effects are delayed, sometimes up to weeks after the medication is started. Homovanillic acid is the major metabolite of dopamine and its levels reflect the dopamine levels in the central nervous system. High levels of this metabolite predict for a positive response to the antipsychotics, since excessive dopamine activity plays a role in the genesis of psychotic symptoms. *(SP 944–945)*

21. Answer is **E.** Electrocardiogram changes may be seen, especially with low-potency agents, and should be thoroughly evaluated since the resulting arrhythmias may be fatal. In general, low-potency antipsychotics are more cardiotoxic than are high-potency agents. *(SP 947)*

22. Answer is **E.** Increased secretion of prolactin results from the blockage of dopamine receptors in the tuberoinfundibular tract and produces a number of unwanted effects. Breast enlargement in men and galactorrhea in both men and women can result. Most distressing are the sexual side effects. Up to 50% of men may experience impotence, and this may have a significant negative influence on compliance. *(SP 948)*

23. Answer is **D.** The bradykinesia, apathy, and masklike facies may be caused by depression, and this possibility should be investigated, as should idiopathic parkinsonism and other possible causes of parkinsonism. Focal perioral tremors (the poorly named "rabbit syndrome") are usually seen late in the course of treatment; other tremors would tend to occur earlier. Amantadine has fewer side effects, but may be less effective in reducing muscle rigidity. Most neuroleptic-induced parkinsonism occurs within the first 90 days of treatment. *(SP 951–952)*

24. Answer is **E.** Perioral, finger, and hand movements are common symptoms of tardive dyskinesia. Stress will exacerbate the movement disorder and the movements vanish with sleep. With 10–20% of patients treated with antipsychotics developing tardive dyskensia after one year of treatment, this problem presents a significant clinical challenge. *(SP 951–952)*

25. Answer is **A.** Mortality rates are especially high with depot agents, perhaps even exceeding 30%. The symptomatology of NMS evolves rapidly, and men generally are affected more than are women. Early symptoms may be mistaken for increased psychosis. Marked body temperature elevation (up to 107° F) can result from NMS, as can elevated blood pressure and pulse. Many laboratory abnormalities are observed with NMS. Leukocytosis increased skeletal muscle fractions of creatinine phosphokinase, and myoglobulinuria with possible renal problems can result. *(SP 953)*

26. Answer is **E.** Antacids and cimetidine can reduce the absorption of antipsychotics if given close to the time of their administration. Toxic levels of diphenylhydantoin can result from phenothiazine inhibition of its metabolism. Thioridazine is especially potent in this regard. Propranolol given in combination with antipsychotics may increase the blood levels of both drugs, resulting in an increase risk of hypotension. Cigarette smoking can reduce plasma levels of antipsychotic drugs, which should be evaluated in patients who smoke. *(SP 954)*

27. Answer is **E.** Antipsychotics have a very favorable therapeutic index, and this may influence clinicians to prescribe excessive dosing. Research indicates that the length of time taken rather than the size of the dose, is most relevant in assessing the efficacy of the medications. Most patients will develop tolerance to side effects while maintaining a positive therapeutic effect. This also may influence the clinician to maintain the patient on a dose that is higher than necessary. Agitation and physical assaultiveness are important symptoms to control in the earliest phase of treatment, however, the use of antipsychotics to sedate patients may result in using too high a dose. Other agents should be employed if sedation or sleep is the desired goal. Staff anxiety about the patient's condition may influence the clinician to use too high a dose to control certain symptoms. gain, it is the length of time on the antipsychotic medication that is the indicator of its effectiveness. *(SP 955)*

28. Answer is **E.** Lithium is rapidly and completely absorbed after ingestion. It is not plasma protein bound and is not metabolized. Lithium crosses the blood–brain barrier slowly, thus making resolution of lithium intoxication a slow process. Like sodium, lithium is reabsorbed in the proximal tubules, being freely filtered at the glomerulus. Lactating women will excrete lithium in breast milk. *(SP 962)*

29. Answer is **E.** Adolescents are usually quite concerned about issues related to body image, and thus may find the adverse effects of acne and weight gain especially troubling. Ebstein's malformation of the tricuspid valve, while a fairly rare event, is quite serious. Lithium should be avoided during pregnancy if possible. If lithium is used during gestation, the lowest possible dose should be given and the lithium level carefully monitored. Changing renal function during pregnancy will influence lithium levels. Lithium's use in geriatric populations is well known. Since the elderly reach a stead-state equilibrium more slowly than do younger people, dosages should be adjusted more slowly. *(SP 965–966)*

30. Answer is **D.** Monamine oxidase is widely distributed with the highest concentrations in the liver, the gastrointestinal tract, the central nervous system, and the sympathetic nervous system. Its primary location is intracellular, located on the external membrane of mitochondria.

Dietary tyramine is deactivated by MAO-A in the gastrointestinal system, and if this enzyme is inhibited, it can enter the circulation and act as a pressor, resulting in a hypertensive crisis. Platelets contain only MAO-B, and thus measurement of its MAO inhibition may not be reflective of brain MAO-A inhibition, the effect most associated with antidepressant activity. The relative specifity of activity of MAO-A and MAO-B has allowed for the development of agents that specifically inhibit one or the other subspecies. *(SP 971)*

31. Answer is **E**. Fluoxetine is metabolized to norfluoxetine, which is active in active in reducing serotonin reuptake and has a longer half-life than does the parent drug. Some patients report excessive stimulation with fluoxetine. Complaints of headaches, nervousness, insomnia, nausea, vomiting, and diarrhea are the most common problems. Sexual dysfunction, such as premature ejaculation, anorgasmia, and impotence, occurs in at least 5% of patients treated with fluoxetine. Fluoxetine does not appear to increase the incidence of fetal abnormalities, although, as with all medications, its use should be avoided during pregnancy. *(SP 978)*

32. Answer is **B**. Alanine aminotransferase is the most sensitive indicator of the hepatic effects of tacrine, and monitoring of this enzyme can be helpful in the detection and prevention of serious hepatic events. The absorption of tacrine is inhibited by food and it should be taken one hour before meals. Its short half-life of three to four hours mandates multiple daily dosing. Thus far, it appears that about 70% of patients will tolerate tacrine for long-term treatment. *(SP 985–986)*

33. Answer is **D**. Like trazodone, the primary action of nefazodone is on serotonin systems. Nefazodone's specific action appears to be antagonism of 5-HT$_2$ receptors and weak inhibition of serotonin reuptake does not seem to play a role in the long-term effects of this drug. Nefazodone has a much more favorable side-effect profile than does trazodone with less sedation and orthostatic hypotension. Priapism also is not a problem with this medication. Two active compounds are produces by nefazodone metabolism. Hydroxynefazodone has an activity profile similar to that of its parent compound. The other metabolite, *M*-chlorophenylpiperazine, is also a metabolite of trazodone and has some postsynaptic serotonin activity. *(SP 990)*

34. Answer is **A**. These drugs are primarily used as antidepressants, however, many other diagnoses, especially Anxiety Disorders, respond well to tricyclic medications. Imipramine is arguably the drug of choice for Panic Disorder. Amitriptyline has a long history of use in the management of chronic pain. Although Bulimia Nervosa and Anorexia Nervosa may respond to tricyclics, obesity may be aggravated by these drugs. *(SP 993)*

35. Answer is **A**. Stopping tricyclic or tetracyclic treatment too soon frequently will result in a reemergence of pretreatment symptomatology. A cholinergic rebound syndrome characterized by nausea, headache, sweating, and neck pain may occur with abrupt cessation of these medications. While these medications do not have addictive risk, a slow taper of 25% reduction the first month and then 25 mg every three days will reduce the likelihood of symptom reemergence or cholinergic rebound syndrome. *(SP 997)*

36. Answer is **D**. Valproate and lithium coadministration will often result in increased tremors, which are effectively treated with beta-adrenergic antagonists. An increased incidence of extrapyramidal events is associated with valproate–antipsychotic combinations, with a resultant increased need for antiparkinsonian agents. Diazepam and phenobarbital levels are increased with valproate coadministration and valproate plasma levels are reduced when coadministered with carbamazepine. *(SP 1002)*

37. Answer is **B**. In addition to a routine physical examination, neurological examination, and preanesthesia examinations, blood chemistries, a chest X-ray, and an ECG should be done on all patients. Spine films should be done on patients who have evidence of spinal abnormality or who may be at special risk for spinal damage, such as elderly women who have osteoporosis. A dental examination is advisable on all patients to assess risk and to assess the status of dentition. Imaging of the brain would be indicated in patient who have evidence of a space-occupying lesion or a suspected seizure disorder. *(SP 1007)*

38. Answer is **E**. Although bilateral placement produces a more rapid response in most patients and in certain conditions, such as severe depression, mania, catatonic stupor, and treatment-resistant Schizophrenia may be indications for a bilateral approach; the usual approach today is to try unilateral placement first. Unilateral placement on the nondominant hemisphere produces less postictal confusion and is preferred when circumstances warrant its use. *(SP 1008)*

39. Answer is **B**. A seizure must last at least 25 seconds to be therapeutic and the clinician should have an objective measure of the seizure activity, most often a single-led EEG. Only rarely does ECT precipitate a seizure disorder in patients. If a particular stimulus fails to produce a seizure, up to four attempts with different settings of stimulus can be tried before the session is terminated. A prolonged seizure is 180 seconds or greater. *(SP 1009)*

40. Answer is **A**. ECT-associated death usually has a cardiovascular cause in patients who have previously compromised cardiovascular systems. Memory impairment has been a chronic concern of clinicians an and patients alike. Patients who experience little improvement from ECT

complain the most about the memory impairment. Many patients will permanently lose their memory for the events leading up to their hospitalization and ECT, but will return to baseline memory function at six months. The mortality rate with ECT is about 0.002% and is much lower than that of the tricyclic antidepressants. It is among the safest somatic treatments in psychiatry when properly administrated. *(SP 1010)*

41. Answer is **b**. Aspirin does not affect lithium levels, although many drugs do. Thiazide and loop diuretics may increase lithium levels. Osmotic diuretics, carbonic anhydrase inhibitors, and xanthines may all reduce lithium levels. Nonsteroidal anti-inflammatory drugs angiotensin–converting enzyme inhibitors cause lithium concentrations to increase. *(SP 966)*

42. Answer is **d**. Lithium levels are drawn 12 hours after the last dose, plus or minus 30 minutes. Lithium may affect the renal, thyroid, and hematopoietic systems, and thus baseline values must be obtained. Women of childbearing years must have a pregnancy test prior to lithium treatment. Most adults can be started at 300 mg three times daily, but the elderly and renally impaired should be started at lower doses. For acute mania, the blood levels should be 1.0–1.5 mEg/L; for maintenance treatment, levels should be 0.6–1.2 mEg/L. While multiple daily dosing is inconvenient, it is still the standard of care. *(SP 967–968)*

43. Answer is **d**. Caffeine should be minimized or eliminated from the diets of patients with tremors. Many psychoactive medications cause tremors, and the tremors will be influenced by the emotional state of the patient. Reduced doses taken at bedtime will help to minimize daytime tremors. *(SP 886)*

44. Answer is **a**. Propranolol is an effective treatment for Acute Akathisia, but not for Acute Dystonia or parkinsonism. This drug may be a useful adjuvant in the treatment of aggressive, violent patients, as well as in Alcohol Withdrawal. Diabetics should not take propranolol because of its blocking physiological responses to hypoglycemia. Some Anxiety Disorders, especially performance-type Social Phobias, may respond quite well to propranolol. *(SP 893–894)*

45. Answer is **c**. Although other agents have eclipsed barbiturates as hypnotics, skillful use of these drugs still has a place in contemporary psychiatric practice. Amobarbital can be used to manage acute agitation in patients, as well as in diagnostic interviews. For barbiturate-addicted patients, the Pentobarbital Challenge Test will safely assess their tolerance, and phenobarbital is the drug of choice for detoxification. *(SP 903)*

46. Answer is **b**. Benzodiazepines are much safer than barbiturates. In overdose situations, benzodiazepines have only a remote chance of a fatal outcome, whereas barbiturates, even with a small overdose, may be fatal. Barbiturates are schedule II drugs, benzodiazepines are scheduled IV drugs, but in New York State, are treated as schedule II drugs. Both have the potential for tolerance and abuse, and they may have seizure activity as a part of their withdrawal patterns. Pregnant women should not receive either of these medications, and women of child bearing age should have a pregnancy test before initiating their use. *(SP 904)*

47. Answer is **a**. All benzodiazepines, with the exception of clorazepate, are absorbed unchanged from the gut. Clorazepate is converted to desmethyldiazepam in the gut and absorbed in that form. All the compounds listed in answer b are the most rapidly absorbed and have the quickest onset of action. The extensive enteroheptic circulation of some benzodiazepines causes a biplasic plasma level curve. While a number of injectable benzodiazepine preparations exist, only lorazepam has been shown to be reliably absorbed from IM injection. The rapidity of absorption and action owes much to the high lipid solubility of benzodiazepines, a characteristic that varies widely in this group of drugs. *(SP 907)*

48. Answer is **e**. While some studies indicate that benzodiazepines my be useful in the treatment of Akathisia when standard treatments fail, the benzodiazepines are not a treatment for dystonic reactions. Anticonvulsant activity is most pronounced with clonazepam. Skeletal muscle relaxation via the inhibition of spinal polysynaptic afferent pathways is a well-known effect of this drug class. Obviously, insomnia and the treatment of Anxiety Disorders are primary uses. *(SP 908–909)*

49. Answer is **b**. Nausea, depersonalization, depression, and perceptual disturbances probably reflect a disordered brain chemistry secondary to a withdrawal syndrome. Headache, especially tension headache, is a frequent complaint in anxious patients, and may represent a return of the original Anxiety Disorder. *(SP 911)*

50. Answer is **c**. The shorter the half-life and the higher the dose, the more severe the withdrawal will be. Longer-half-life benzodiazepines entail a less severe withdrawal because their blood levels fall more slowly. Even with a controlled taper of not more than 25% per week, most patients will experience some form of withdrawal. Some clinicians have found low-dose carbamazepine (400–500 mg a day) to be useful and supportive psychotherapy that can help patients better address the withdrawal phase. *(SP 912)*

51. Answer is **d**. Zolpidem has no active metabolites and is not chemically related to the benzodiazepines. Its affinity is much greater for the $BZ_1$ receptors of the central nervous system giving it potent hypnotic effects, but no skeletal muscle or anxiolytic properties. Tolerance and

dependence have not been reported with this medication. *(SP 914)*

52. Answer is **a**. Carbamazepine is well known to suppress WBC levels. Usually the WBCs rebound toward normal, and this initial suppression has a benign course, however, rarely, carbamazepine results in serious marrow suppression. The cause of this phenomenon is thought to be an inhibition of colony-stimulating factor, and lithium does reverse this effect. Carbamazepine does have a vasopressin-like effect that causes hyponatremia with a particular sensitivity to this effect seen in the elderly. Another endocrine effect is an increase in urinary free cortisol. Atrioventricular conduction is decreased by carbamazepine, limiting its use in patients with A-V blocks. *(SP 926–927)*

53. Answer is **c**. Gastrointestinal distress, with nausea, vomiting, and diarrhea, are the most common side effects of carbamazepine administration. Elderly and cognitively impaired patients may experience the most CNS toxicity from carbamazepine. Typically. drowsiness, confusion, ataxia, and tremor are the most common adverse effects. The benign WBC suppression seen early in carbamazepine treatment does not correlate with the more serious potentially life-threatening blood dyscrasias. Hepatic hypersensitivity is a serious adverse effect, and may result in death if the drug is reintroduced in a patient with this reaction. Pregnant women should not take carbamazepine unless absolutely necessary since significant fetal abnormality may result. *(SP 926)*

54. Answer is **b**. The most serious adverse reactions to carbamazepine involve the hematological, hepatic, and cardiac systems, and any preexisting conditions should be thoroughly evaluated. Allergic hypersensitivity to tricyclics should be evaluated since carbamazepine is structurally related to the tricyclics, especially imipramine. Twice-monthly CBCs for the first two months and then quarterly CBCs are no longer recommended by the FDA. Hematological monitoring is left to the discretion of the physician. This conservative monitoring schedule is not cost effective and is not particularly effective in its protection from an adverse hematological event. Carbamazepine may be started at 200 mg twice daily, increased by 200 mg every 2 to 4 days, up to an average dose of 1,000 mg a day. Plasma levels can be monitored and the oral dose should yield a plasma level of 4 to 12 µg/ml. This drug may be discontinued abruptly without problems. *(SP 929)*

55. Answer is **b**. Dystonic reactions and other parkinsonian effects rarely occur with clozapine. Patients taking more than 600 mg per day have a seizure rate of about 5%. This is a dose-related effect and decreases with a decrease in the dose. However, the seizure incidence is higher than with standard antipsychotics. Sedation and drowsiness may be especially troubling to patients. Bone marrow suppression is a well-known adverse effect of clozapine, occurring in 1–2% of patients. Most often, it occurs within six months of initiation of treatment but may arise much later. Increased age and being female increase the risk. Tachycardia, hypotension, and electrocardiogram change all occur with clozapine. *(SP 934)*

56. Answer is **c**. Although the tricyclic compounds' antidepressant effects require weeks to develop, the inhibiting effects on the monoamine reuptake pump occurs within minutes of the first dose. Amitriptyline is a tertiary amine, as are imipramine and doxepin. Side effects are generally more pronounced with the tertiary amines than with the secondary amines. Like most antidepressants (and electroconvulsive therapy) tricyclics cause a down-regulation of central beta-adrenergic receptors. The significance of this finding is unknown since not all antidepressants cause the phenomenon. Tricyclic antidepressants have no effect on the synthesis of monoamines. *(SP 991–992)*

57. Answer is **a**. Tertiary amines more potentially inhibit the reuptake of serotonin. The first-pass metabolites—the secondary amines—more potentially inhibit the reuptake of norepinephrine. Thus, TCAs have a dual effect. Orthostatic hypotension is a frequent undesirable side effect of TCA treatment caused by peripheral beta-adrenergic blockade, not anticholinergic activity. Dry mouth, urinary retention, constipation, dry eyes, etc., result from anticholinergic blockade. The unwanted weight gain is associated with the TCA's antihistamine activity. Tricyclics exert a quinidinelike effect on cardiac conduction and arrhythmia and the life-threatening sequelae of an overdose, not respiratory depression. *(SP 991–998)*

58. Answer is **d**. Two subtypes of monoamine oxidase, MAO-A and MAO-B have been identified. The reuptake pump is the predominant means of removal of amines from the synapse. MAO is intracellular as well, both in the cytosol and associated with mitochondria. MAO-A deaminates norepinephrine and serotonin and MAO-B primarily deaminates dopamine, although both subtypes contribute to the metabolism of dopamine. *(SP 971–972)*

59. Answer is **e**. The risk of seizures with bupropion treatment is two to four times greater than with other antidepressants. The risk is especially great with oral doses of more than 150 mg at one time or total daily doses exceeding 400 mg. At therapeutic levels the other antidepressants are not as strongly associated with seizure activity. *(SP 919)*

60. Answer is **d**. Bupropion and amphetamine share the characteristic of blocking the dopamine reuptake pump, but only amphetamine is taken up by the pump and stored in vesicles. Bupropion's structure is similar to that of dopamine, does not affect other neurotransmitter systems, and is not addictive. *(SP 919)*

**61.** Answer is **b**. Bupropion is not associated with nausea. The selective serotonin reuptake inhibitors' most frequently reported side effect is nausea. It is also a common side effect of the novel antidepressant venlafaxine. *(SP 919, 978, 980–981, 1003)*

**62.** Answer is **b**. Aphasia is characteristic of cortical dementias such as Dementia of the Alzheimer's Type but not of subcortical dementias such as HIV-related dementia. Balance problems with rapid head turns are quite common and may place the patient at some risk for physical injury. Dementia Due to HIV Disease most typically is a late event in the course of the illness and has a classic triad of cognitive, behavioral, and motor problems. These patients may become very withdrawn and amotivational late in the course of the disease process. *(SP 378–379)*

**63.** Answer is **e**. Adjustment Disorders are the most common diagnosis in the HIV-positive population. Depression, dementia, and substance abuse are also common diagnoses. Sexual dysfunction may also occur early in the course of the illness, mostly due to psychological issues as well as later in the course of the illness as a result of medications and the effects of dealing with chronic medical illness. *(SP 380)*

**64.** Answer is **d**. Oral doses represent the average doses that produce a maximal positive result and a minimal negative result. The GI absorption is essential for delivering drug to the bloodstream, and patients do not universally absorb drugs with the same efficiency. The blood flow to a particular part of the brain, the blood–brain barrier, and the receptor's affinity for the drug are all important in the ultimate distribution of the medication to the brain. *(SP 866–867)*

**65.** Answer is **e**. Orthostatic hypotension results from alpha-adrenergic blockage. The others listed are a result of acetylcholine blockade. *(SP 873)*

**66.** Answer is **c**. An intense initial phase of CNS stimulation characterized by confusion, agitation, hallucinations, hypertension, hyperreflexia, and seizures is followed by CNS depression with hyperthermia, areflexia, respiratory depression, and cardiac conduction abnormalities. *(SP 880)*

**67.** Answer is **b**. This ECG finding may be the best overall predictor of the severity of the overdose. Hyperreflexia, respiratory depression, decreased bowel sounds, and a positive response to physostigmine may all be present, but may not be indicative of the seriousness of the overdose. The cardiac conductive effects of tricyclics are well known and they represent a major threat to the patient's life in an overdose situation. *(SP 880)*

**68.** Answer is **d**. Being female increases the risk of developing Neuroleptic-Induced Tardive Dyskinesia, as do the other factors listed. *(SP 885)*

**69.** Answer is **c**. Lithium does not bind to plasma proteins and is not metabolized. It is distributed throughout total body water, however, this is a nonuniform distribution. Lithium, either in normal doses or in an overdose situation, does not readily cross the blood–brain barrier. This explains why lithium intoxication may take much time to resolve. Lithium is almost entirely excreted by the kidneys, with most of it being absorbed by proximal tubules. *(SP 962)*

**70.** Answer is **a**. Lithium blocks the release of thyroid hormone from the thyroid gland, and thus can result in hypothyroidism and goiter. Lithium can influence the action of antidiuretic hormone on the distal tubules of the kidneys, resulting in a nephrogenic diabetes insipidus. Some patients must avoid lithium because of its effect on sinus node function. The thyroid effects of lithium are seen more frequently in women. *(SP 964–965)*

**71.** Answer is **e**. Lithium maintenance should be seriously considered for patients who have a strong history of Bipolar I Disorder since these patients are especially at risk. The lack of precipitating factors for the first episode and high suicide risk are also strong indicators for lithium maintenance. If the patient is 30 years of age or older, has a sudden onset of a first episode, and is male, these are also strong reasons to maintain the patient on lithium. Data indicate that patients who are initially responsive to lithium but fail to take their lithium or were not maintained on lithium lost their lithium responsiveness with subsequent episodes. *(SP 962–963)*

**72.** Answer is **b**. Tremor is a common finding, occurring in 50% or more of lithium-treated patients. It is most notable in the outstretched hands, and especially in the fingers. The tremor can be worse during peak drug levels, and propranolol in low doses often will provide complete resolution of the symptom. Clinicians should be alert to this side effect as it may compromise compliance. *(SP 964)*

**73.** Answer is **d**. Lithium antagonizes the action of antidiuretic hormone on the distal renal tubules, resulting in a nephrogenic diabetes insipidus and polyuria. A large percentage of lithium-treated patients have this problem (25–35%). Dehydration can result, and patients with the problem must be carefully monitored. Treatment with a thiazide diuretic may help, but the lithium dose must be halved to compensate for lithium retention with this medication. Originally, lithium was thought to be quite nephrotoxic but now the renal sequelae of long-term lithium administration seem to be less than was believed to be the case. *(SP 964)*

**74.** Answer is **b**. Propylthiouracil, sulfonamides, and captopril are all associated with bone marrow suppression or agranulocytosis, and such medications should not be coadministered with clozapine. The benzodiazepines may aggravate the orthostatic hypotension and resultant syncope, as well as rarely causing respiratory depression. Other CNS depressants, alcohol, and TCAs may put the patient at risk for seizures, sedation, and cardiac effects. Coadministration of lithium also may increase the seizure risk, confusion, and movement disorders. A few case reports suggest that lithium not be used in conjunction with clozapine in patients who have experienced the Neuroleptic Malignant Syndrome. *(SP 935)*

75. Answer is **b**. Usually, clozapine may be started at 25 mg once or twice a day and gradually increased to minimize adverse effects, such as hypotension, syncope, and sedation. The usual effective treatment range is 400–500 mg/day, although some patients may require up to 600 mg/day. One milligram of clozapine is equivalent to 1.5–2 mg of chlorpromazine. When deciding to terminate the drug, a tapering schedule will help to avoid the development of rebound cholinergic symptoms. *(SP 935)*

76. Answer is **d**. Disulfiram increases the blood concentration of many medications, including diazepam, phenytoin, anticoagulants, and tricyclic drugs. It is very well absorbed from the GI tract, is metabolized by the liver, and is renally excreted. By a pronounced inhibition of alcohol dehydrogenase, blood levels of aldehyde markedly increase after alcohol ingestion, producing the unpleasant reaction for which disulfiram is so well known. Severe alcohol–disulfiram reactions are a medical emergency that requires prompt intervention, as cardiorespiratory collapse, seizures, and death may result. Disulfiram may be a useful adjuvant to a comprehensive treatment plan for the treatment of Alcohol Use Disorders, but all patients on disulfiram should be closely monitored. *(SP 937)*

77. Answer is **a**. All of the effects listed can be caused by antipsychotics, especially low-potency agents, with the exception of reduced coronary artery blood flow. *(SP 945)*

78. Answer is **c**. A transient leukopenia may result from the administration of antipsychotics, and rarely agranulocytosis may occur. Skin rashes, photosensitivity, and discoloration may also be observed, although infrequently. Sexual dysfunction occurs quite commonly in both men and women, and often plays a role in noncompliance. Vasodilation and orthostatis due to alpha-adrenergic blockade are also common occurrences. *(SP 945)*

79. Answer is **d**. Less than a quarter of patients with Schizophrenia maintained on antipsychotic medications relapse during the first year of treatment, and these relapses are less severe than the symptoms of patients not receiving these medications. Generally, the positive symptoms of Schizophrenia, such as agitation, hallucinations and delusions, are most responsive to antipsychotic med-

ications. Negative symptoms, such as isolation, withdrawal, and apathy may not respond to these medications and may worsen under their influence. Paranoid patients have numerous positive symptoms, and thus may respond better than will nonparanoid patients. *(SP 945–946)*

80. Answer is **c**. Agranulocytosis usually occurs within the first three months of treatment. A benign, usually transient, leukopenia may be commonly observed. Routine CBC monitoring is not recommended, although fever, sore throat, and other symptoms of a compromised immune system should be immediately evaluated. The incidence of agranulocytosis is five per 10,000 and the mortality rate may be as high as 30%. *(SP 948)*

81. Answer is **c**. Thioridazine in doses exceeding 800 mg can result in irreversible retina damage and blindness. The pigmentation of the retina may proceed even after the medication is withheld and is similar to that of retinitis pigmentosa. In contrast, chlorpromazine can produce granular deposits in the anterior lens and posterior cornea, visible only with slit lamp examination. At times, these patients may have a brownish discoloration of the conjunctiva. Retinal damage is not seen with chlorpromazine, and the eye changes are seen only in patients who have been taking chlorpromazine for many years. *(SP 949)*

82. Answer is **c**. Women are twice as likely as men to develop Neuroleptic-Induced Parkinsonism, which most commonly develops after the age of 40. About 15% of all patients treated with neuroleptics develop parkinsonism. Symptoms include muscle stiffness, cogwheel rigidity, shuffling gait, and stooped posture. A true pill-rolling tremor is rare, although other tremors may be present. A positive physical sign of parkinsonism is a positive glabella tap reflex, which is characterized by a failure of the orbicularis oculi to habituate to repeated taps between the eyebrows. Although antipsychotics can cause this parkinsonism, the highpotency/low-anticholinergic medications may cause the most problems. Blockade of dopaminergic pathways in the nigrostriatal tract causes this clinical situation. *(SP 949)*

83. Answer is **e**. Dopaminergic hyperactivity in the basal ganglia as CNS levels of antipsychotic medications fall between doses has been postulated as a possible cause of dystonia. Most dystonic reactions will occur promptly with the initiation of treatment, an exception being the oculogyric crisis, which may occur late in treatment. Children are especially likely to experience opisthotonos, scoliosis, lordosis, and writhing movements. Dystonia is most frequently seen in men under the age of 40. These involuntary movements frequently are painful and frightening, and may sharply decrease compliance. The potential benefits of prophylaxis with anticholinergic agents should be considered. *(SP 950)*

84. Answer is **a**. Recent studies have challenged the notion that Tardive Dyskinesia is always chronic and progressive. It tends to develop rapidly, stabilize, and frequently remit, even when the medication continues uninterrupted. Between 5% and 40% of all cases remit, and in mild cases, up to 90% may remit. Prevention is the key in addressing the problem of Tardive Dyskinesia. Accurate diagnosis and a treatment plan focused on target symptoms using the lowest dose of antipsychotic possible are important. Clinicians should conduct regular, objective evaluations of patients at risk for Tardive Dyskinesia and document their findings. Dopaminergic receptors in the basal ganglia are believed to be rendered supersensitive to dopamine, with chronic blockade. *(SP 951–952)*

85. Answer is **b**. Although not all antipsychotics lower the seizure threshold, some do, and careful evaluation of patient's seizure history is important. Narrow-angle glaucoma may worsen when the patient is exposed to antipsychotics. Tardive Dyskinesia may also worsen with reexposure to an antipsychotic, however, a careful analysis of the potential risks and benefits should be done on a case-by-case basis. With some antipsychotics, any known cardiac abnormalities must be thoroughly assessed before instituting pharmacotherapy. *(SP 955)*

86. Answer is **d**. Lithium impedes the release of thyroid hormone from the thyroid, resulting in a rise in thyroid-stimulating hormone. Many patients experience polyuria adverse effects from chronic lithium administration. The mechanism of action is antagonism of antidiuretic hormone in the distal tubules of the kidney. Gastrointestinal complaints are very frequent with lithium administration, and can be reduced by giving lithium with meals, in slow-release preparations, and at a lower dosage. Benign T-wave flattening or inversion is the most common finding on the ECG of lithium-treated patients. Such changes disappear when lithium is discontinued. Lithium is known to cause a leukocytosis from its stimulation of colony-stimulating factor. *(SP 964–965)*

87. Answer is **a**. Weight gain, edema, and sexual dysfunction usually do not respond to treatment and require a change to another medication. Rarely, the MAOI alone in the absence of tyramine can cause a hypertensive crisis. Most frequently, however, the most common cardiovascular effect is hypotension. Hepatotoxicity may result from phenelzine and isocarboxazid. Over-the-counter decongestants, especially those containing dextromethoraphan, must not be used by patients on MAOIs. *(SP 972–973)*

88. Answer is **c**. Tricyclic medications can be safely mixed with fluoxetine at low doses. It can be safely used with warfarin and with sympathomimetics. With the long half-life and its metabolite, norfluoxetine, five weeks must elapse between the cessation of fluoxetine and the initiation of a MAOI. These long half-lives also account for the slow development of a steady-state equilibrium. *(SP 978–979)*

89. Answer is **d**. Dextroamphetamine is rapidly metabolized, with a half-life of only six hours. Dosing is thus multiple times a day. The release of dopamine, and to some extent norepinephrine, is the central action of sympathomimetics. These drugs also inhibit the monoamine reuptake pump, and monoamine oxidase to some degree. The net result is a pronounced dopaminergic response. Long-term use or abuse of these agents results in tolerance to the euphoric and sympathomimetic effects, although not to the therapeutic effects. Sympathomimetics can be used in combination with antidepressants, especially in refractory patients. The metabolism of tri- and tetracyclic drugs is inhibited by sympathomimetics, and increased plasma levels result. *(SP 981–982)*

90. Answer is **e**. Of patients treated with tacrine, 25% to 30% have elevated liver enzymes, and hepatoxicity must be carefully monitored and evaluated. Tacrine inhibits acetylcholinesterase, which is its therapeutic action in mildly to moderately affected Alzheimer's patients. Gastrointestinal distress can result from its muscarinic activity in the parasympathetic nervous system. *(SP 985–986)*

91. Answer is **a**. Trazodone has no anticholinergic activity, and thus avoids many of the adverse reactions of the tricyclic drugs. Its half-life is 6–11 hours, with its primary metabolism in the liver. Priapism, while rare, is a potential problem with trazodone. The drug should be promptly stopped and a urological consultation must be considered if the priapism persists. With its marked sedative qualities and favorable effect on sleep architecture, trazodone is widely used as a hypnotic. *(SP 989–990)*

92. Answer is **b**. Tricyclics are not completely absorbed after oral administration. After absorption, they are tightly bound to plasma proteins and their half-lives vary widely. Many tricyclics (and other drugs) are metabolized by the hepatic enzyme $P_{450}IID6$. Perhaps 8–10% of caucasians are "poor metabolizers" and may have increased effects from these medications. Percentages of poor metabolizers in other racial groups are unknown at present. Many tricyclics are transformed by first-pass metabolism from tertiary amines into secondary amines, which are active compounds. These secondary amines have significantly different therapeutic and adverse effects from the parent compound. *(SP 991–992)*

93. Answer is **e**. Doxepin is the most antihistaminic of this group of drugs. Although the inhibition of the reuptake of biogenic amines occurs within minutes to hours of an oral dose, an antidepressant effect is delayed for weeks. The down-regulation of beta-adrenergic and $5-HT_2$ receptors has been postulated to play a role in this process. However, some effective antidepressants (e.g., paroxe-

tine) lack this effect, so the mechanism of antidepressant action remains unknown. *(SP 992)*

94. Answer is **a**. The antihistaminic effects account for the sedative effects of the tricyclic medications. Anticholinergic effects are common, but some degree of tolerance will usually develop with time. Orthostatic hypotension is the most common side effect and can affect patients of all age groups, not just elderly patients. Imipramine has a pronounced quinidinelike effect on cardiac conduction, which can be exploited when using this drug in cardiac patients, but this should be done only in consultation with a cardiologist. Weight gain is a troublesome and common side effect of the TCAs and is attributable to the blockade of the histamine type 2 receptors. *(SP 993–994)*

95. Answer is **b**. Plasma levels of both tricyclic and tetracyclic drugs may be increased by their coadministration. These medications may also interfere with antihypertensive medications, such as blocking the neuronal uptake of guanethidine, and the effects of beta-adrenergic antagonists. Oral contraceptives may induce hepatic enzymes and then reduce plasma levels of tricyclic and tetracyclic drugs as a result of increased metabolism. The sedative effects of CNS depressants may be magnified if these drugs are taken with tricyclic and tetracyclic drugs. *(SP 995)*

96. Answer is **c**. As with so many medications, GI upset is relatively common. Aside from this effect, valproate is quite safe and only rarely causes serious hepatoxicity or pancreatitis. Carbamazepine and valproate are not chemically related, although both are used to treat similar psychiatric conditions. Valproate's actions are poorly understood but seem linked to GABA systems, not the noradrenergic system of the locus ceruleus. Weight gain may be a problem with maintenance of a patient on this medication. Use in pregnancy should be avoided because of possible neural tube defects in the fetus (e.g., spina bifida). *(SP 1000–1001)*

97. Answer is **a**. Venlafaxine may act more promptly to relieve depressive symptoms than other antidepressants and shows promise in treating more severely depressed patients. Its short half-life of five hours requires twice or three times a day dosing. At higher doses (375 mg or more per day), about 3% of patients experience elevated blood pressure. Venlafaxine nonspecifically inhibits the reuptake of norepinephrine, serotonin, and dopamine, while having no effects on muscarinic, histaminic, or adrenergic receptors. Venlafaxine is metabolized in the liver and has at least one active metabolite. *(SP 1003–1004)*

98. Answer is **d**. Seventy percent of patients receiving ECT have a diagnosis of Bipolar Disorder. Major Depressive Disorder, Manic Episodes, and in some cases Schizophrenia are indications for ECT. Occasionally, Obsessive-Compulsive Disorder and Catatonic Disorder will be treated with ECT when other treatments fail. *(SP 1006)*

99. Answer is **a**. Tricyclics, tetracyclics, MAOIs, and antipsychotics are generally acceptable in a patient undergoing ECT. Clozapine should be discontinued because it is associated with the appearance of late-appearing seizures, Benzodiazepines should be withdrawn because of their anticonvulsant activity. Lithium may contribute to the development of a postictal delirium and prolonged seizure activity. Theophylline may increase the duration of the seizures. *(SP 1007)*

100. Answer is **a**. A 40-fold variability exists in patients in regard to seizure threshold; ECT itself causes a rise in the seizure threshold. The elderly and men have higher thresholds than do women and young adults. Most clinicians will initiate ECT by selecting an electrical stimulus that is judged to be subthreshold and increasing that value by 100% for unilateral electrode placement and by 50% for bilateral electrode placement. *(SP 1008)*

101. Answer is **c**. Patients with Catatonic Disorder may respond to as few as one to four treatments. Usually, ECT is given two to three times weekly, with the twice-weekly schedule resulting in fewer memory problems. The usual course of treatment is six to 12 sessions, but in some cases, up to 20 sessions may be required. The patient must be carefully monitored to observe for continued improvement and any side effects. Maximal therapeutic value is defined as when the patient fails to improve after two consecutive treatments. Before ECT is abandoned, a trial of bilateral, high-intensity ECT should be given. *(SP 1009)*

102. Answer is **b**. Fetal monitoring is not required in uncomplicated normal pregnancies. There are no absolute contraindications to ECT, but special consideration must be given in certain clinical situations. Patients who have had a recent myocardial infarction are a high-risk population, but research indicates that after two weeks the risk becomes substantially less. After three months, the risk is even further reduced. Patients with hypertension should be stabilized on their medications before beginning ECT. Space-occupying lesions in the cranium pose a risk of edema and herniation. Some clinicians recommend pretreatment with dexamethasone and controlling the hypertension during the seizure as an approach to dealing with this situation. *(SP 1010)*

103. Answer is **c**. Phototherapy is still under active investigation, but it seems that morning exposure for approximately one hour with light that is 200 times brighter than normal indoor illumination is an effective treatment for Mood Disorder With Seasonal Pattern. Thirty minutes of exposure would be too brief for most patients to benefit. *(SP 1011)*

# 4

# SELECTED TOPICS

# QUESTIONS

**DIRECTIONS: For questions 1 through 16, select the single best answer.**

1. All of the following statements about compliance are correct **EXCEPT**:

    a. Compliance is improved when the patient continues to see the same physician.
    b. Compliance is better in patients with more chronic illness.
    c. Compliance is less in patients who are in a multiple-dose regimen.
    d. Poor compliance may be a direct expression of psychopathology.
    e. Compliance is improved with a good doctor–patient relationship.

2. All of the following statements about Postpartum Psychosis are correct **EXCEPT**:

    a. Peak incidence occurs during first two weeks postpartum.
    b. Over 80% are diagnosed as Mood Disorder.
    c. Prophylactic chemotherapy prevents recurrence in most cases.
    d. Frequently these patients have obsessive thoughts of harming the infant.
    e. Most recover from acute episode.

3. All of the following are examples of tertiary prevention **EXCEPT**:

    a. Group homes
    b. Social skills training
    c. Genetic counseling
    d. Home visits to monitor medication
    e. Assistance with income support programs

4. All of the following statements about the impaired physician are correct **EXCEPT**:

    a. Colleagues tend to deny and cover up the problem.
    b. Frequently the physician denies having a problem.
    c. Once the physician starts treatment, he or she is likely to persist.
    d. Suicide risk is higher in male physicians as compared with female colleagues.
    e. Psychiatrists have a significantly higher risk of Mood Disorder.

5. All of the following statements about the psychiatrist expert witness are correct **EXCEPT**:

    a. It is unethical to agree on a fee dependent on the trial settlement.
    b. It is unethical to rehearse testimony before the court

    appearance.
    c. Psychiatrist has to answer questions even if disadvantageous to his or her client.
    d. The judge decides whether the psychiatrist is a qualified expert.
    e. The expert is not obliged to answer with "Yes" or "No" when asked.

6. Recent court decisions regarding involuntary commitment have set the standard of proof of dangerousness as:

    a. 95% certainty
    b. 75% certainty
    c. 51% certainty
    d. 40% certainty
    e. $33^1/_3$% certainty

7. All of the following statements about involuntary commitment are correct **EXCEPT**:

    a. Commitment is a legal decision.
    b. Commitment has to be to a hospital setting.
    c. Commitment usually has a time limit.
    d. Commitment is based on the parens patriae principle.
    e. Commitment does not require the permission of responsible relatives.

8. As a result of the California court rulings in the Tarasoff case, many states have now changed their laws regarding the clinician and:

    a. Criminal responsibility
    b. Threats against a third party
    c. Involuntary commitment
    d. Alleged sexual abuse of children
    e. Use of hearsay evidence

9. In situations of spouse abuse, all of the following are correct **EXCEPT**:

    a. Abusing spouse was likely to have been an abused child.
    b. Abused spouse was likely to have been an abused child.
    c. Spouse abuse is highly related to drug abuse and alcoholism.
    d. Pregnancy tends to protect against abuse.
    e. Abused husbands fear ridicule if they expose the problem.

10. In an initial interview, a young male patient becomes increasingly agitated and eventually starts toying with a nasty looking knife. The clinician, in this situation, could reasonably adhere to any of the following procedures **EXCEPT**:

    a. Leave the office and call the security staff.

b. Offer food to the patient.

c. Ask the patient if he wishes medication.

d. Ask the patient what is troubling him.

e. Insist that the patient hand over the weapon.

11. When a college graduate is asked the meaning of the proverb "People who live in glass houses should not throw stones," her response is, "You might get cut by the glass." Her reply shows:

a. Autistic thinking

b. Illogical thinking

c. Concrete thinking

d. Magical thinking

e. Abstract thinking

12. A Type I error occurs when:

a. A null hypothesis is retained when it should have been rejected.

b. A null hypothesis is rejected when it should have been retained.

c. The construct validity is not established.

d. The sample study is not drawn properly.

e. The correlation coefficient is low.

13. According to a null hypothesis:

a. The testing instrument does not measure what it was designed to measure.

b. The risk factor does not precede the disability.

c. The observed differences can be explained by chance alone.

d. The probability rating is zero.

14. When a patient scores markedly lower on block design and picture arrangement subtests than on verbal performance tests in the Wechsler Intelligence Scale, these results suggest:

a. Damage to nondominant hemisphere

b. Major Depressive Disorder

c. Malingering

d. Chronic undifferentiated Schizophrenia

e. Psychogenic amnesia

15. A 35-year-old man, right-handed and moderately aphasic, scores 78 on the verbal scale and 99 on the performance scale of the Wechsler Adult Intelligence Scale. These test results would support the diagnosis of:

a. Left hemisphere damage

b. Bilateral parietal lobe lesions

c. Right hemisphere damage

d. Diffuse cerebral deterioration

e. Conversion Disorder

16. In the National Institute of Mental Health (NIMH) Epidemiologic Catchment Area survey, the most common disorder, according to one-month prevalence, was:

a. Obsessive-Compulsive Disorder

b. Phobia

c. Dysthymic Disorder

d. Alcohol Dependence

e. Substance Dependence

For questions 17 through 59, one or more of the alternatives may be correct. After deciding which of the alternatives is correct, record your answer according to the following key.

A. Alternatives 1, 2, and 3 are correct.

B. Alternatives 1 and 3 are correct.

C. Alternatives 2 and 4 are correct.

D. Alternative 4 only is correct.

E. All four alternatives are correct.

17. Which of the following would be appropriate procedures in an involuntary admission?

1. The patient is discharged from the hospital because he refused to consent to a specific treatment.

2. The patient is committed because she refused to take medication voluntarily.

3. As part of the total treatment, the doctor refused to write to the Social Security office until the patient signed the consent form.

4. Because the patient was dangerous to herself, she was legally committed and medicated.

18. Which of the following statements about the mentally retarded in North America are correct?

1. The majority have mild mental retardation.

2. The highest incidence of diagnosed retardation is found in adolescence.

3. Most are not diagnosed until they attend school.

4. Most eventually require institutional care.

19. Examples of secondary prevention include:

1. Establishment of emergency psychiatric clinics

2. Establishment of halfway houses

3. Mandated mental health insurance coverage

4. Vocational rehabilitation programs

20. Examples of primary prevention include:

1. Education about AIDS for high school students

2. Repainting of inner-city houses

3. Alcohol abstinence during pregnancy

4. Establishment of crisis hotline

21. On which of the following occasions is privileged communication waived?

1. On the decision of the patient

2. On the decision of the physician

3. When the patient is suing the doctor

4. On the decision of the patient's lawyer

22. Which of the following statements about medical privilege is/are correct?

1. A patient has the right to prevent the doctor from giving information.
2. The doctor is obligated to keep information in confidence.
3. Privilege is waived when a patient's mental status is at issue.
4. The physician decides whether to exercise privilege.

23. Which of the following statements apply to the legal doctrine *Respondeat Superior*?

    1. The psychiatrist is legally responsible for the actions of the resident he or she supervises.
    2. The consultant is usually responsible for the clinical results of the treatment recommended.
    3. The clinician is obliged to make sure that his or her supervisees live up to accepted psychiatric standards.
    4. The paternal powers of the state over its citizens are defined.

24. Which of the following statements about psychiatric expert witnesses is/are correct?

    1. A resident in training cannot be an expert witness.
    2. Board certification is required for an expert witness.
    3. An expert witness can only comment on direct observations of the case.
    4. Testimony of an expert witness may include hearsay evidence.

25. The criteria for testamentary capacity include which of the following?

    1. Knowledge of one's possessions
    2. Knowledge of the natural heirs who would expect to receive bequests
    3. Recognition that one is making a will
    4. Absence of psychotic thinking

26. For a patient to give informed consent, which of the following is/are applicable?

    1. The patient is told about the risks and the benefits of the proposed treatment.
    2. The patient must give consent willingly and freely.
    3. The patient knows the alternative treatments possible.
    4. The patient understands the results of no treatment.

27. For a person to be considered competent to stand trial, which of the following should be demonstrated?

    1. Ability to read charges and evidence
    2. Ability to consult with his or her attorney
    3. Ability to know right from wrong
    4. Ability to understand the charges

28. Under the M'Naghten rule, which of the following findings would indicate that the individual was not criminally responsible?

    1. The individual was involuntarily committed to a psychiatric hospital.

2. The individual did not know that the criminal behavior was bad.
3. The individual was mentally retarded.
4. The individual did not understand what he or she was doing.

29. Which of the following statements are correct regarding the M'Naghten rule?

    1. It is a definition of criminal responsibility.
    2. It is primarily a test of cognitive functioning.
    3. It does not take into account the emotional factors.
    4. It focuses on the ability to control impulses.

30. The statement of the American Psychiatric Association on the insanity defense makes which of the following points?

    1. Recommends the possible diagnosis of "guilty but mentally ill."
    2. Sets out clear guidelines for prediction of dangerousness.
    3. Urges reinstatement of the Durham rule.
    4. Recommends that psychiatrists evaluate only the patient's mental state.

31. Which of the following statements about battered spouses is/are correct?

    1. Pregnancy usually produces a reduction in abuse.
    2. Problem is much more common among lower socio-economic groups.
    3. Abusing husband usually does not abuse children.
    4. Abused wives very often were abused as children.

32. In the management of a potentially violent patient, the clinician should use which of the following techniques?

    1. Always look the patient directly in the eye.
    2. Reassure the patient with a gentle pat on the shoulder.
    3. Interpret the reasons for the patient's feeling.
    4. Speak in a soft, nonchallenging fashion.

33. If a patient produces a gun during an interview, the clinician should take which of the following steps?

    1. Take the gun from the patient.
    2. Ask the patient to drop the gun on the floor.
    3. Try to ignore the gun and focus on what the patient is saying.
    4. Ask the patient to put the gun on the desk.

34. Appropriate indications for the use of physical restraints would include which of the following?

    1. Racial insults directed toward staff
    2. Retarded patients threatening other patients
    3. Punishment for repeated stealing from other patients
    4. Delirium of unknown etiology

35. Which of the following statements apply to men who have been raped?

    1. They often fear they will become homosexual.
    2. They are likely to have Posttraumatic Stress Disorder symptoms.

3. They frequently experience sexual dysfunction following rape.
4. The feeling of guilt is common.

36. In the management of a female rape victim, which of the following procedures is/are appropriate:

1. To support the patient in forgetting the trauma
2. To assist in reporting the assault to the police
3. To investigate previous sexual behaviors
4. To refer to rape victim group therapy

37. Female rape victims are likely to experience:

1. Recurrent shame
2. Feelings of defilement
3. Fear of male friends
4. Ruminations about the assault

38. The appropriate emergency management of the female rape victim would include:

1. Detailed assault report in the patient's own words
2. Prophylactic treatment for gonorrhea
3. Collection of pubic hair and vaginal smear specimens
4. Delayed emotional ventilation until female clinician is available

39. Which of the following statements are true about the NIMH Diagnostic Interview Schedule?

1. It is formulated to allow computer scoring.
2. It is derived from the Schedule for Affective Disorders and Schizophrenia.
3. The questions are to be read exactly as worded.
4. It is developed for nonclinician administration.

40. Which of the following statements are true about the Present State Interview?

1. It is used in international studies.
2. It deals mainly with psychoses.
3. It requires specially trained interviewers.
4. It gathers detailed long-range data.

41. Short-term memory can be tested by:

1. Having the patient draw pictures of figures after these figures have been removed from view
2. Asking what the patient had for breakfast, when one knows the menu
3. Asking the patient to recall five digits reversed
4. Asking the patient to name the first president of the United States

42. Which of the following statements about IQ scores on the Wechsler Adult Intelligence Scale are correct?

1. Sixty-eight percent of the population have IQs in the range of 85 to 115.
2. The average IQ is 85 to 100.
3. An IQ of 110 is at the 75th percentile level.
4. Seven percent of the population have IQs of 70 or below.

43. In using the Wechsler Adult Intelligence Scale, early senile dementia should be suspected in a patient where:

1. Both visual and performance scores are lower than premorbid ability.
2. The performance scale is significantly below verbal scale score.
3. The person is unable to construct blocks to conform to a picture design.
4. The person scores low on similarities subtest.

44. Serial 7's Test is characterized by which of the following statements?

1. It is affected by patient's motivation.
2. It measures ability to maintain attention.
3. It is impaired by thought disorder.
4. Errors may indicate depression.

45. Correct statements about the Draw-A-Person Test include:

1. It is a projective test for personality assessment.
2. It is an intelligence test for children.
3. It can be used to detect brain damage.
4. It affords better validation than most projective tests.

46. When the Bender Gestalt Test is used for psychological evaluation, which of the following suggest brain damage?

1. Language deficits
2. Perseveration
3. Color shock
4. Incomplete angulation

47. Which of the following statements about the Bender Gestalt Test is/are correct?

1. Designs may be directly copied.
2. Poor motivation may give false positive results.
3. Rotation of figures indicates organicity.
4. Differentiates Delusional Disorders Due to a Medical Condition from Schizophrenia.

48. Which of the following statements about the Rorschach test are true?

1. It has ten ambiguous inkblots.
2. Each presents black, gray, white, and colored stimuli.
3. It sets no limit on number of responses.
4. It is a useful, well-validated research test.

49. When the Rorschach test is used to evaluate a patient, which of the following is/are significant?

1. The degree to which the patient reacts to the color in the blots.
2. The patient's perception of the actual shape of a blot.
3. The content of the patient's response.
4. The patient's recognition of deviant responses.

50. The Rorschach test of an emotionally withdrawn patient will usually demonstrate:

1. Poor form level
2. Preoccupation with shades of black and gray

3. Bizarre content
4. Few color responses

51. Which of the following statements about the L, F, and K Scales of the Minnesota Multiphasic Inventory is/are correct?

    1. Useful in identifying malingering
    2. Evaluates attitude toward test-taking
    3. Indicates invalid test if unduly elevated
    4. May be elevated with illiteracy

52. Which of the following statements about the Minnesota Multiphasic Inventory is/are true?

    1. Has a series of true or false questions
    2. May be computer scored
    3. Is the most widely researched personality test
    4. Individual clinical scales are specifically diagnostic

53. Which of the following statements about the Thematic Apperception Test are correct?

    1. It is made up of a series of black, white, and colored pictures.
    2. It requires the patient to construct a story.
    3. It is computer scored.
    4. It portrays people in ambiguous situations.

54. Which of the following responses on the Rorschach test would support the diagnosis of Schizophrenia?

    1. Inability to integrate color into perception
    2. Poor form responses
    3. Contamination of responses
    4. Very limited popular responses

55. In the NIMH Epidemiological Catchment Area Program, studies showed:

    1. Obsessive-Compulsive Disorder higher in men than women
    2. Phobia more common in females than males

3. Depression more common over age 65 than between ages of 25 and 44
4. Schizophrenia diagnosed equally in men and women

56. When a test group is said to have normal distribution, which of the following statements would be correct?

    1. Sixty-eight percent of the group lie within two standard deviations of the mean.
    2. The median and the mode are equal.
    3. The variance is the square root of the standard deviation.
    4. The mean and the median are equal.

57. In experimental design, which of the following statements is/are correct?

    1. In normal distribution, two standard deviations from the mean covers 95% of the population.
    2. A Type I statistical error occurs when a null hypothesis is inappropriately retained.
    3. A kappa level of 0.80 indicates higher rater agreement.
    4. With a normal distribution, the variance and the standard deviation are equal.

58. In a research study, which of the following statements are correct?

    1. The independent variable is controlled by the researcher.
    2. The dependent variable is the focus of the study.
    3. The incidence rate is the rate of new cases occurring within a specific time.
    4. ANOVA compares different sets of findings.

59. Which of the following statements about the Global Assessment of Functioning Scale is/are correct?

    1. Rating made for the past six months
    2. Rating 20 would indicate danger to self or others or severe impairment
    3. Includes impairment due to social, physical, and environmental factors
    4. Used on Axis V of DSM-IV

# ANSWERS AND EXPLANATIONS

1. Answer is **b**. Compliance, also called adherence, is the degree to which a patient carries out prescribed treatment. In general, one third of patients comply, one third sometimes comply, and one third do not. There is no association of compliance with the patient's age, sex, marital state, race, or demographic characteristics. Compliance is increased by the physician's characteristics of enthusiasm, permissiveness, age, experience, time spent with the patient, a short waiting time, and the doctor–patient relationship ("match"). Communication is important for the physician for the treatment, the names of drugs and their side effects, an understanding of the illness, and any compromises made in treatment (patient contract).

    Compliance is decreased if the patient has to take more than three different types of medications and must take them more often than four times a day, utilizing purely verbal instruction if side effects are present; if beneficial effects have slow onset; if the patient has financial hardships or a lack of confidence in treatment; or if multiple clinicians are involved. Psychiatric patients have a higher degree of noncompliance than do medical patients. *(SP 11–12)*

2. Answer is **c**. About 40–50% of women report "postpartum blues," which is an emotional disturbance or cognitive dysfunction experienced in the postpartum period. Postpartum psychosis is rare, occurring in one to two per 1,000 deliveries. Most patients with postpartum psychosis have an underlying mental illness, particularly Bipolar Disorder, and less often, Schizophrenia. A premorbid history of marital problems is also a major factor. Postpartum psychosis occurs usually about the third postpartum day, and most cases are seen within 30 days. *(SP 36, 494–496)*

3. Answer is **c**. Tertiary prevention is the reduction of the prevalence of a residual defect or disability due to an illness or disorder. It involves rehabilitative efforts to enable those who have a chronic illness, mental or physical, to reach their highest level of functioning feasible. Included in tertiary prevention is a broad range of services, such as inpatient, outpatient, and supervised living arrangements; peer, family, and community support systems; case management; and social and vocational rehabilitation. *(SP 203)*

4. Answer is **d**. Doctors disabled by alcohol or drugs are often difficult to detect, owing both to the conspiracy of silence surrounding them and their own self-deception. Characteristic behaviors of impaired physicians are, first, they withdraw from the community and friends; next, they change jobs, often repeatedly; then their physical status begins to deteriorate; and, finally, they no longer can func-

tion effectively at the office and in the hospital. Those who are involved in rehabilitation programs have a reported 73–97% success rate. *(SP 1193–1194)*

5. Answer is **b**. More and more often the psychiatrist is playing a major role as an expert witness. Rarely is the psychiatrist "independent" but is selected for one of the sides in a case. Direct examination is given by the attorney representing the party on whose behalf the witness is called. It is "friendly" and has been rehearsed before the trial. *(SP 1171–1172)*

6. Answer is **b**. Involuntary commitment permits hospitalization against a patient's will, is based on the principles of the "parens patriae" (father of the country) and the "police power" of the state, and is justified by an individual's inability to make decisions in his or her own best interest and the need to protect the individual from himself or herself.

    The minimal legal standard of proof in civil commitment cases is "clear and convincing" of 75% sure, rather than the stricter "beyond a reasonable doubt" of 90% sure for criminal guilt. In civil suits, a "preponderance of the evidence" is based on over 50% certainty and is required for liability. Hearsay is often admissible for involuntary commitment procedures. *(SP 1176)*

7. Answer is **b**. Mental health codes' civil commitment laws detail patient's right to treatment and right to refuse treatment. Regulation of commitment is predominantly through statutory law (based on the parens patriae and police power) rather than case law. Two legal principles protect all patients against involuntary treatment. The first, from common law, states that a doctor who treats a patient without consent, except under special circumstances (emergency), will be guilty of battery (illegal touching), and the second lays forth that a doctor who treats a patient without informed consent, except under special circumstances, is guilty of negligence.

    The right to treatment is still unsettled in many jurisdictions. The constitutional significance was recognized in *Wyatt v. Stickney* (1972), which held: "To deprive any citizen of his or her liberty upon the altruistic theory that the confinement is for humane and therapeutic reasons and then fails to provide adequate treatment violates the very fundamentals of due process." In 1982 (*Romero v. Youngberg*), the U.S. Supreme Court ruled that the "right to habilitation" was a narrow right to treatment for the institutionalized mentally retarded. *(SP 1176–1178)*

8. Answer is **b**. The Tarasoff case (*Tarasoff v. Regents of the University of California*, 1976) set a standard that applies

to a physician or a psychotherapist who has reason to believe that a patient may injure or kill someone. The professional must notify the potential victim, his or her relatives or friends, and the authorities. (SP 1174)

9. Answer is **d**. Wife beating occurs in all cultures and in all types of families. Substance abuse plays a major role. The Surgeon General identified pregnancy as high-risk period for battering; 15 to 25% of pregnant women are physically abused and this often results in birth defects. (SP 793)

10. Answer is **e**. Offices should not contain heavy throwable objects such as ashtrays, but should contain pillows or a light chair, which can be used as a shield or protection. The clinician should communicate in a neutral concrete manner about the obvious, such as, "You look angry. Could you tell me what you are concerned about?" The physician should appear calm and in control and speak softly in a nonprovocative and nonjudgmental manner. Undue direct eye-to-eye contact should be avoided. Medications or food can be offered. Continue to evaluate by asking questions. (SP 812–813)

11. Answer is **c**. The thought content of a patient's thinking can be assessed through responses to various questions obtained during an evaluation. Thought process is the flow of ideas, symbols, and associations. Normal thinking is directed toward a reality-oriented conclusion in a logical sequence.

Autistic thinking has no regard for reality and reveals preoccupations with an inner, private world.

Illogical thinking contains erroneous conclusions or internal contradictions.

Concrete thinking is literal and one-dimensional thought with a limited use of metaphors.

Magical thinking refers to a form of dereistic thought, similar to the preoperational phase in children (Piaget) in which thoughts, words, or actions assume power.

Abstract thinking is the ability to appreciate nuances of meaning and is multidimensional with the ability to use metaphors and hypotheses appropriately. (SP 813–814)

12. Answer is **b**. Type I and Type II errors are two types of potential errors that can occur in a research or statistical study. A Type I error occurs when the null hypothesis is rejected or declared false when it should have been retained or is true. A Type II error occurs when the null hypothesis is retained as true when it should be rejected or is false. (SP 199)

13. Answer is **c**. The null hypothesis is the assumption that there is no significant difference between two random samples of a population. The null hypothesis also states that observed differences or variations in scores can be attributed to random sources. When the null hypothesis is rejected, observed differences between groups are deemed to be improbable by change alone. (SP 199)

14. Answer is **a**. The Wechsler Adult Intelligence Scale—Revised (WAIS-R) contains about 80% of the WAIS from the Wechsler-Bellevue series of standardized intelligence tests. There are 11 subtests: six in the verbal scale (V)—information, comprehension, arithmetic, similarities, digit span, and vocabulary; and five in the performance scale (P)—digit symbol, picture completion, block design, picture arrangement, and object assembly. Generally, the difference between the V and P scales is less than 15 points. Disproportionate impairment in the verbal scale as compared with the performance scale is primarily associated with left (dominant) hemisphere damage and aphasia.

A right (nondominant) hemisphere impairment shows relatively normal verbal scale scores, but marked impairment in the performance scale. A parietal lobe impairment in either hemisphere results overall in a lower performance scale. This pattern is also seen in diffuse cerebral disturbances or in multifocal damage, such as with a head injury or a dementia. A full-scale (FS) decrease (because of both verbal and performance lower scores) is seen with depression, poor motivation, and cerebral disease. (SP 1157)

15. Answer is **a**. Impaired intellectual functioning often accompanies cerebrovascular disease and brain tumors. The WAIS reflects such psychopathology. (SP 368)

16. Answer is **b**. The NIMH Epidemiologic Catchment Area (ECA) survey provides the most complete data about the prevalence of mental disorders in persons of all ages. Results of this study show that about 15.4% of the general U.S. population had one or more DSM-IV disorders one month before the interview (14% males compared with 16.6% females). Eleven and one-half percent (11.5%) of the population had a substance-use problem.

Prevalence rates of other current disorders were: Schizophrenia 0.7% (males equal females); Affective (Mood) Disorders 5.1% (males 6.6%, females 3.5%); Anxiety Disorders (the highest prevalence) 7.3% (females 9.7%, much greater than in males 4.7%); Phobias (had the greatest increase from prior studies) 6.2%; Substance Use Disorder 3.8% (males 6.3%, females 1.6%); Somatization Disorder 0.2% (almost all females); Antisocial Personality Disorder 0.5% (males 0.8% and females 0.2%); severe Cognitive Disorder 1.3% (males equal to females). (SP 194–196)

17. Answer is **D**. Involuntary admission is based on evidence that the patient is a danger to himself or herself (i.e., suicidal) or a danger to others (homicidal), gravely disabled, and more recently, a substance abuser. An involuntary admission request may be made by a relative, a friend, or the police, depending on various state laws. In most states, usually two physicians can hospitalize a patient for up to 60 days, but the patient must have access to legal counsel and a judge to review the case. The patient has a right to file a petition for a writ of habeas corpus by himself or

herself, or it can be done by others if it is believed that the patient has been deprived illegally of liberty. Each state has its own standards and procedures for voluntary and involuntary entry into a mental hospital. *(SP 1176)*

18. Answer is **A**. Up to 85% of the mentally retarded population fall in the mild category. *(SP 1025)*

19. Answer is **B**. Secondary prevention is defined as the early identification and prompt treatment of an illness or disorder with the goal of reducing the prevalence (total number of existing cases) or severity of the condition. The military principles of treatment reference "PIE" (Proximity, Immediacy, and Expectancy) could be applied to civilian programs. Included in secondary prevention strategies are emergency services, outpatient services, day treatment, community-based inpatient units, removal of economic barrier to treatment, insurance, and prepaid health plans. *(SP 203)*

20. Answer is **A**. Primary prevention is the prevention of the onset of a disease or disorder, thereby reducing its incidence (number of new cases occurring in a specific period). Primary prevention strategies include the elimination of etiological agents and reduction of risk factors through mental health education, efforts at competence building, development and utilization of social support systems, and establishment of anticipatory guidance programs to assist in crisis intervention after stressful events, such as death, marital separation, and group disasters. Other areas of primary prevention include reducing stress during prenatal and perinatal care through proper diet, adhering to lead pollution laws, and genetic counseling. *(SP 203)*

21. Answer is **B**. Privileged communication refers to the rights of patients that certain confidential information not be disclosed in a judicial setting. Privilege belongs to the patient, not to the physician.

    Confidentiality concerns the communication of private information from one person to another under conditions that the recipient of information will not ordinarily disclose the information to a third person. Confidentiality is limited by legal statute (Tarasoff rule).

    Privacy refers to limiting the access of others to one's body or mind, including dreams, fantasies, thought, or beliefs, and is linked to freedom from intrusion by the state or third persons. *(SP 1172–1173)*

22. Answer is **B**. Patient information must be kept confidential unless the patient releases the psychiatrist from professional secrecy or a vital common value in the patient's best interest makes disclosure imperative. The patient must be informed of the breach of secrecy. *(SP 1172–1173)*

23. Answer is **B**. The legal doctrine of *Respondeat Superior*

refers to a physician who supervises another (supervisee) and is responsible both ethically and legally for the quality of the services delivered, due to the actual or apparent control exercised over the supervisee. The supervisor must ensure the patient be informed of such a relationship. *(SP 1184–1185)*

24. Answer is **D**. An expert witness provides psychiatric facts or opinions that are relevant to the ultimate legal determination. The expert is required to identify the medical and psychiatric data that are applicable to the existence of a psychiatric disorder and is expected to relate these data to the legal definition of a standard of criminal responsibility. *(SP 1171–1173)*

25. Answer is **A**. Competency to make a will is called "testamentary capacity" and cognitive capacity is emphasized. Three psychological abilities are required. Individuals must know (1) the nature and extent of their bounty (property), (2) that they are making a will, and (3) who their natural beneficiaries are. Some additional factors may be used, such as having sufficient mind and memory to understand those facts, the ability to recall the decision that was formed, and the ability to appreciate the relationship of the facts to one another. *(SP 1179–1180)*

26. Answer is **E**. In general, informed consent requires the following criteria or data: (1) an understanding of the nature and foreseeable risks (side effects) and benefits of a procedure; (2) knowledge of alternative procedures; (3) an awareness of the consequences of withholding consent; (4) the recognition that the consent is voluntary (no coercion, explicit or implicit); and (5) having the legal capacity to give consent (i.e., adult), and if not, must be given by a relative or court-appointed guardian. The data should be documented in writing or on a special form. *(SP 1178–1179, 1191–1192)*

27. Answer is **C**. The test of competency to stand trial is set either by statute or case law and may be worded differently in different jurisdictions. Essentially, competency to stand trial is a two-pronged test involving the capacity to consult with one's lawyer and the ability to understand the proceedings against one. It says nothing of the patient's overall mental competency or functioning. *(SP 1180)*

28. Answer is **C**. The M'Naghten rule (1843) stated that every man is presumed to be sane, and in order to be considered insane it must be clearly proved that the accused was laboring under such a defect of reason, from disease of the mind, as not to know that what he was doing was wrong. *(SP 1181)*

29. Answer is **A**. The M'Naghten rule emphasized cognitive defects and eliminated the requirement to prove frenzy and lack of volitional control. It ignored emotional derangement or loss of volitional control. *(SP 1181)*

30. Answer is **D**. In 1982 Congress adopted the definition of insanity based on the American Psychiatric Association and American Bar Association recommendations as to whether the defendant, as a result of mental disease or defect (mental illness) was unable to appreciate the nature and quality of the wrongfulness of his or her conduct (acts), and that "mental illness" was to be limited to a "severely abnormal" mental condition (meaning psychosis). *(SP 1180–1183)*

31. Answer is **D**. Spouse abuse is a severe problem seen in every racial and religious group and in all socioeconomic strata. It is more frequent in families of drug abusers, particularly of those who abuse alcohol. Men who abuse their spouses generally come from violent homes where they witnessed wife beating or were abused themselves as children. As husbands, they tend to be immature, dependent, and nonassertive, and to suffer from strong feelings of inadequacy. Wife abuse is most common, but some husbands are abused. Husband abuse is underreported, as the men fear ridicule if they expose the problem, a counterassault, or loss of financial support. *(SP 793)*

32. Answer is **D**. Violence and assaultive behavior in a patient are very difficult to predict. The best predictors are excessive alcohol intake; history of violent acts, with arrests or criminal activity; and a history of childhood abuse. Violent patients are often frightened by their own hostile impulses and desperately seek help to prevent loss of control. Management of a violent patient is by physical means; restraints should be applied if there is a reasonable risk of violence. The patient should be approached with sufficient help and with overwhelming strength, so that there is no contest.

    Violent, struggling patients may be effectively subdued with appropriate sedative or antipsychotic medication: diazepam (Valium) 5–10 mg intravenously (IV), or lorazepam (Ativan) 2–4 mg intramuscularly (IM) or IV, haloperidol 5–10 mg IM, or chlorpromazine 25–50 mg IM. The clinician should appear calm and in control, sit if possible, and not tower over the patient. The psychiatrist should listen to the patient and assess the potential for violence, as indicated by threats, availability of means, and history. *(SP 812–813, 815–816)*

33. Answer is **D**. Safety is the first concern if there is a danger to the therapist. There should be some way to communicate the danger to others, such as by a buzzer, code words, or other prearranged signals. If the patient has a gun, one should comply with requests if one cannot escape. The patient should be asked to put the gun on a desk and not to drop it or throw it, as it may discharge. Armed police officers should always remove bullets from their weapons while in the emergency room, ward, or clinic. *(SP 812–813, 815–816)*

34. Answer is **C**. Emergency seclusion and restraints are used to prevent imminent harm to others or to the patient if other means are not effective or appropriate, to prevent serious disruption of the treatment program or damage to environment (as part of an ongoing behavior treatment program), to decrease stimulation of the patient, and on the patient's request (seclusion). There must be a written policy with specific guidance for the staff on the use of seclusion and restraints, with ongoing education and reviews. *(SP 812–813, 815–816)*

35. Answer is **E**. Women who are raped experience shame, humiliation, confusion, fear, and rage, lasting a year or longer. Posttraumatic Stress Disorder, phobia of sexual interactions, and vaginismus are common sequelae. Male rape is legally defined as sodomy. Homosexual rape is more frequent with men. Men feel similar to women who were raped, and also feel they "have been ruined," and some fear they will become homosexuals. *(SP 793, 795)*

36. Answer is **C**. Treatment of rape victims is most effective with immediate support, where the victim is able to ventilate her feelings and rage to loving family members, sympathetic physicians, and supportive law enforcement officials. If the victim knows she has a socially acceptable means of recourse at her disposal, such as the arrest and conviction of the rapist, this will be therapeutic. Supportive therapy, especially group therapy with homogeneous groups composed of rape victims, is usually beneficial. *(SP 793, 795)*

37. Answer is **E**. All too often society sees the rape victim as less a victim but perhaps guilty of provoking the rape! The result is that the victim feels shame and anger that often leads to clinical depression. *(SP 793–795)*

38. Answer is **A**. Rape crisis centers and telephone hotlines are available for immediate aid and information for victims. There are legal requirements for the collection of specimens such as pubic hair and vaginal smears, to determine the presence of spermatozoa. Trauma to the skin or body or other activities should be carefully documented, with photographs if possible. A detailed report of the incident in the patient's own words should be made as soon as possible in order to prevent later distortions. Prophylactic treatment for venereal disease, such as gonorrhea, is important. (SP 793–795)

39. Answer is **E**. The NIMH Diagnostic Interview Schedule (DIS) was designed for epidemiological studies of general populations. It combines the Research Diagnostic Interview (RDI) and the Schedule for Affective Disorders and Schizophrenia (SADS). Epidemiologists developed fully structured interviews, according to DSM-IV criteria, to be used by nonclinicians to access a large number of subjects. Exact wording is used in each question, with a "Yes"

or "No" answer. Problems are coded by condition, not by psychiatric illness. The system uses a computer program to score the information and to make diagnostic assignments. The DIS results assess the occurrence of symptoms at any time in the patient's life. *(SP 194)*

40. Answer is **A**. The Present State Examination (PSE) measures the current mental state of a patient and is intended for use by skilled clinicians who are trained in the administration of the test and who must demonstrate adequate levels of interrelater reliability.

    The interview form concentrates mainly on psychotic conditions. Its primary aim was to compare rates of Schizophrenia in international studies, and it covers only the one-month state prior to the interview. Historical information is not obtained. PSE results do not give diagnostic labels according to any established classification system. *(SP 196)*

41. Answer is **A**. Memory functions have been traditionally divided into four types: immediate, recent, recent past, and remote. Immediate and recent memories, also called short-term memory, consist of less than five minutes for recent recall, and have a capacity limited to about seven, plus or minus two, chunks (or alternatives) of information.

    Recent past and remote memories, also called long-term memory, are the retention of experiences over hours or days for recent past memory, whereas remote memory goes to earlier life. Long-term memory involves consolidation of information into a relatively permanent store that subsequently is retrievable.*(SP 170, 231)*

42. Answer is **B**. The Wechsler Adult Intelligence Scale is designed so that the average performance (average IQ) is a mean of 100 with a standard deviation of 15 points. In addition, norms have been constructed for different age ranges, so that a subject's IQ can be compared with an age-matched comparison group. Sixty-eight percent of the population have an IQ of 85-115 (one standard deviation). Ninety-five percent of the population have an IQ of 70-130 (two standard deviations). *(SP 222–223)*

43. Answer is **E**. The Wechsler Adult Intelligence Scale (WAIS) and the WAIS-R have a full-scale score (FS) and two major scales, verbal scale (VS) and performance scale (PS) scores. The verbal scale reflects retention of previously acquired (and frequently overlearned) factual information. There are six subtests: information, comprehension, similarities, arithmetic, digit span, vocabulary.

    The performance scale measures visuospatial capacity and visuomotor abilities. There are five subtests: digit symbols, picture completion, picture arrangement, block design, object assembly. When the performance scale IQ is significantly lower than the verbal scale IQ, this is a useful indicator of cerebral damage. *(SP 222–223)*

44. Answer is **E**. Attention and concentration of cognitive

functioning can be tested by four tests: Serial 7's, the "A" test, Digit Span, and Spelling Backwards. The Serial 7's test consists of taking 7 from 100 and 7 from each remainder. It requires rudimentary subtraction ability and measures the patient's ability to sustain the task in mind and keep track of sequential answers.

    The "A" Test consists of the patient's tapping his or her finger every time the examiner says "A'." Most individuals can immediately repeat a digit span of at least five digits forward and four digits in reverse order. Most can spell a five-letter word forward and then backwards. Errors in any of these tests may occur because of poor motivation, delirium, dementia, depression, psychosis, or mental retardation. *(SP 337)*

45. Answer is **A**. Draw-A-Person (DAP) or figure drawings can be classified as projective tests as they allow individuals to project interpersonal psychic and familial conflicts or their own personality onto the drawings. DAP scoring procedures are available for the estimation of intelligence and are mostly used with the mentally retarded or with children. A manual is available for dynamic and analytically oriented interpretation of the figure drawings, but such data lack validity. *(SP 229)*

46. Answer is **C**. The Bender Gestalt Test consists of nine geometric figures. Some clinicians use the copied figures as a projective test and try to infer personality characteristics, but this use is of questionable validity. The Bender Gestalt Test is primarily used as a graphic test for constructional praxis in adults and children since it measures visuoconstructive ability. It can also be used to test memory by waiting 45–60 seconds before having the patient copy the figures from memory. The Bender Gestalt Test is helpful in testing for brain damage, where patients are likely to show perseverations, problems with incomplete angulations and juxtaposition, and a tendency to verticalize diagonals and to substitute loops for dots. *(SP 1037, 1157)*

47. Answer is **A**. The Bender Gestalt (Visual Motor) Test can be used from ages 3 to 4 years to any older age. There are nine separate designs copied directly on paper. A patient's poor motivation may result in false positives. The rotation of copied figures may indicate organicity. *(SP 1037, 1157)*

48. Answer is **B**. The Rorschach (inkblot) test is an unstructured, projective test using 10 plates of ambiguous inkblots. The patient's responses are scored on multiple criteria referencing accuracy of form, movement, and location, and use of color, shading, and details; these scores are put into three general coded categories of location, determinants, and form quality content. The test provides information on a patient's level of functioning, maturity, reality testing, interpersonal relations, and emo-

tional responsiveness. It can be helpful in the evaluation of psychosis, suicidality, depression, and anxiety problems. *(SP 227, 229, 1022–1023)*

49. The answer is **E**. The Rorschach results are coded in the following important categories:

Location—what portion of blot is utilized

Determinants—aspects of blot salient to the patient's perception of form, color, shading, and movement

Form content—the specific character of the perception that is human, animal, or nature *(SP 227–229, 1122–1123)*

50. Answer is **D**. Rorschach responses of an emotionally withdrawn patient will usually be limited in number, with an avoidance of color responses and with unimaginative observations. *(SP 227–229, 1122–1123)*

51. Answer is **E**. The questions involved in the Minnesota Multiphasic Personality Inventory (MMPI) were developed from lists of psychiatric symptoms and complaints and various published personality inventories. The MMPI is a self-report, paper-and-pencil test consisting of a series of 550 true–false (T-F) items. The data are shown via three validity scales and 10 standard clinical scales based on norms obtained from large pools of psychiatric and non-psychiatric clinical patients. The MMPI is set up to assess possible malingering.

The major strength of the MMPI is that it is the most widely used and researched psychological test. Computerized scoring is available. There is a shorter version of the test that consists of 90 items and is used for screening. *(SP 223–226)*

52. Answer is **A**. The original MMPI appeared in the late 1930s and is the most thoroughly researched and used examination for personality assessment. Its newest updated version is the MMPI-2. The test scores 10 standard clinical scales. The newest version is based on a contemporary sample of normal people and questions have been updated to reflect current cultural views. *(SP 223–226)*

53. Answer is **C**. The Thematic Apperception Test (TAT) started out as a study of normal personalities, but has evolved into a projective test used in psychological examinations. There are 30 cards with pictures varying in content, containing one or more characters, and having various degrees of ambiguity. However, only 10–12 cards tend to be used because of time limitations.

Information is obtained from responses regarding the patient's beliefs, needs, traits, attitudes, and motives—in general, a broad spectrum of behavior and cognition. Standardized scoring does exist, but most interpretation is impressionistic and informal. *(SP 229)*

54. Answer is **E**. The Rorschach test is of limited value in

diagnosing Schizophrenia. However, both the Rorschach and TAT responses from psychotic patients generally reveal bizarre ideation. In the Rorschach responses, there is likely to be confabulation and contamination; poorly perceived form responses; repetitions of one concept; a lack of imagination, movement, and human content; and an inability to integrate color into the percepts. Overall, there are usually fewer responses and popular observations are often absent. *(SP 227–228)*

55. Answer is **C**. A major goal of the NIMH-ECA was to determine specifically the prevalence of mental disorders as defined by DSM-III-R and eventually DSM-IV. *(SP 194–195)*

56. Answer is **B**. In a test group, the normal distribution is the mean, median, and mode, and these will be the same when the distribution of scores is normal. The median is the halfway point or 50th percentile in the distribution. The mode is the most frequent (common) score in the distribution. The mean is the arithmetic average and is important in determining the standard deviation. The standard deviation (SD) is a mathematical measure of the spread of scores clustered about the mean. In a normal distribution, 65% of the measurements lie within one SD of the mean, and 95% will be within two SDs of the mean. *(SP 194–195)*

57. Answer is **B**. In a population experimental design, a normal distribution consists of 95% of individuals or two standard deviations from the average. Kappa ($\kappa$) is the most widely used measure of agreement for reliability that corrects for the proportion of chance agreements. Guidelines for interpreting kappa are that values above 0.75 are excellent, 0.40–0.75 are good, and below 0.40 are poor. The value depends on how common the particular condition is in the study sample. *(SP 197)*

58. Answer is **B**. Analysis of variance (ANOVA) is a set of statistical procedures designed to compare two or more groups of observation. The independent variable is studied in relation to an outcome or dependent variable. In experiments, the independent variable is controlled by the experimenter. The dependent variable is the phenomenon of interest in a research study and is also called the outcome variable. The incidence rate is the rate at which new cases of a disease or a condition are occurring within a defined period and is usually expressed as a number per 1,000. *(SP197)*

59. Answer is **D**. The Global Assessment of Functioning (GAF) is on Axis V of the DSM-IV Multiaxial System of classification of diagnostic criteria. The summary of the five axes is as follows:

Axis I—Clinical syndromes to include the V codes.

Axis II—Personality and developmental disorders.

Axis III—Existing medical or physical disorders or conditions.

Axis IV—Severity of psychosocial stressors that are relevant to the illness. The rating scale is a continuum of 1 (no stressors) to 6 (catastrophic), and 0 (inadequate information or no change) codes.

Axis V—GAF Scale. The highest level of functioning exhibited during the previous year (social, occupational, and psychological functioning). There is a scale of 1–90, with 1–10 (grossly impaired) to 90 (absent or minimal symptoms, good functioning in all areas) and 0 (inadequate information). *(SP 317–318, DSM-IV 32–33)*

# 5
## CASE
## HISTORIES

# QUESTIONS

**DIRECTIONS: For questions 1 through 16, select the single best answer.**

*1–6.* Helen, who is 17 years old, was brought in by her parents because of significant weight loss. Helen denies having any feeling of physical hunger and states that she continues to have a normal lifestyle and level of physical activity.

1. What would you most expect to find in your clinical examination of Helen?

   a. Hyperproteinemia
   b. Normal skin tone
   c. Diarrhea
   d. Amenorrhea
   e. Hyperkalemia

2. Your differential diagnosis at this stage would include all of the following except:

   a. Hypothyroidism
   b. Chronic disease, especially granulomatosis disease of the small bowel
   c. Neoplasms
   d. Occult infections
   e. Primary or secondary Depressive Disorder

3. Assuming your diagnosis is Anorexia Nervosa, what is most characteristic of Helen's history?

   a. Normal growth and development
   b. Ability to talk about her feelings
   c. A strong sense of independence from her mother
   d. Onset after a strenuous attempt at dieting
   e. No early feeding problems

4. What would most influence your decision to hospitalize Helen?

   a. All patients diagnosed with Anorexia Nervosa must be hospitalized.
   b. Denial by patient that she has a problem
   c. Lack of awareness or distorted self-concept
   d. Pregnancy fantasies
   e. Body weight below 50% of ideal weight

5. If Helen is not hospitalized, what issue is most important for her outpatient treatment?

   a. Placement on psychotropic medication
   b. Close communication among patient, her family, and the professional staff
   c. Group psychotherapy for Helen
   d. Dietary record keeping
   e. Family therapy

6. If Helen requires hospitalization, what is the least concern you might have in your discharge plans?

   a. Placement of Helen out of the home
   b. Follow-up treatment team that includes the pediatrician and psychiatrist
   c. Public health nurse support
   d. School placement
   e. Ongoing communication among all parties involved in Helen's treatment

*7–16.* Beth is a 14-year-old girl who was hospitalized on the pediatric ward after her diabetes got out of control and she developed ketoacidosis. The request from pediatrics for psychiatric consultation states: "Patient is a management problem. Please advise."

7. Based on this limited information, your first step should be to:

   a. Send the consult request form back with a note to the effect that there is insufficient information.
   b. Read the patient's chart.
   c. Talk to the nurses on the floor where the patient is hospitalized.
   d. Call the referring pediatrician and ask for more information about the request.
   e. See the patient.

8. You learn that Beth was first diagnosed as having juvenile onset diabetes mellitus in childhood and was under good control until she entered adolescence, when she became noncompliant with diet, urine checks, and dosage adjustments. She has been in the hospital five times in the past year with severe ketoacidosis. Based on this, the most likely explanation for her behavior is:

   a. Her diabetes has become more difficult to control as a result of hormonal variations.
   b. The frequent episodes of ketoacidosis represent disguised suicide attempts.
   c. Her difficulty in controlling her diabetes represents a struggle with tasks of adolescent development.
   d. Her physician is mismanaging her.
   e. Beth has a psychiatric disorder.

9. You learn that Beth has markedly decreased potassium and increased serum amylase on a regular basis. When you mention this to her attending, she says that she suspects that the patient may be vomiting. The patient is 5 feet, 5 inches tall, and she weighs 90 pounds. The most likely diagnosis in the following differential is:

   a. Bulimia Nervosa
   b. Anorexia Nervosa
   c. Prader-Willi syndrome

d. Psychogenic vomiting

e. Generalized Anxiety Disorder

10. Additional evaluation leads you to believe that the patient has Bulimia Nervosa and is self-inducing vomiting. When you share this with the attending, she becomes very angry at the patient for "causing" her own life-threatening illness. Which of the following interactions with the pediatrician is likely to be the least helpful to Beth in the long run?

a. Offering to take over the management of the case

b. Offering to be part of Beth's treatment team on pediatrics

c. Explaining the developmental nature of Beth's disorder

d. Offering clear suggestions for working effectively with Beth

e. Determining the source of the pediatrician's anger

11. The nursing staff members on the floor where Beth is hospitalized are divided in their opinions of Beth: some like her very much and defend her, and the others are very angry with her and critical of her. Which of the following suggestions is likely to be the least helpful to Beth and the nursing staff?

a. Designating a team of nurses to work with Beth

b. Instituting a postmeal watch with a nurse and Beth

c. Meeting daily with the team of nurses working with Beth

d. Pointing out to the nurses that their anger at or defense of Beth has to do with their own control issues

e. Providing the nursing staff with reading material about eating disorders

12. You meet with Beth's parents. Her father is a successful politician in the community, and is often away from the home. Her mother is an attorney who stopped practicing several years earlier so that she could be at home with Beth. You sense that there is a great deal of marital conflict, and that is causing Beth distress. Which of the following is likely to be the least helpful suggestion to the parents?

a. Suggesting another meeting with the family while Beth is in the hospital

b. Suggesting that they give their permission to talk with the family doctor in order to gather further information

c. Suggesting that the mother go to work and that the father spend more time at home

d. Suggesting that the family may benefit from family therapy

e. Suggesting to the family that emotional stress can exacerbate physical disorders

13. In your fourth meeting with Beth, she confides in you that her father has been sexually molesting her for several months. The molestation consists of genital fondling in her bed late at night and has not involved penetration.

Which of the following possible actions is the most appropriate?

a. Notify the authorities immediately.

b. Notify the attending pediatrician immediately to determine who will notify the authorities.

c. Gather further information before notifying the authorities.

d. Insist that the father have no further contact with Beth.

e. Continue the evaluation without notifying the authorities since penetration did not occur.

14. Based on this new information, Beth is at risk of having or developing all of the following disorders. Which is the least likely?

a. Posttraumatic Stress Disorder (PTSD)

b. Somatization Disorder

c. Substance Abuse

d. Major Depressive Disorder

e. Conduct Disorder

15. Which of the following considerations is the least importantin considering whether and when to arrange for Beth to be transferred to a psychiatric unit?

a. Beth's medical condition is stable enough to be managed on the psychiatric unit.

b. The psychiatric unit agrees to manage Beth's medical condition.

c. Beth agrees to the transfer to the psychiatric unit.

d. The parents agree to the transfer to the psychiatric unit.

e. The attending pediatrician agrees to the transfer to the psychiatric unit.

16. Based on the combination of Beth's disorders, which of the following is the most likely prognosis?

a. Beth will not have significant psychiatric difficulties in the future.

b. Beth will be overly concerned with food and weight and her sexuality, but will live a fairly "normal" life.

c. Beth will have episodic psychiatric disability during times of stress and is at increased risk of depressive disorders.

d. Beth will have chronic psychiatric disability and is at increased risk of suicide.

e. It is too early to say for certain whether Beth will do well or do poorly.

DIRECTIONS: For questions 17 through 51, one or more of the alternatives may be correct.After deciding which of the alternatives is correct, record your answer according to the following key.

A. Alternatives 1, 2, and 3 are correct.

B. Alternatives 1 and 3 are correct.

C. Alternatives 2 and 4 are correct.

D. Alternative 4 only is correct.

E. All four alternatives are correct.

*17–18.* The distraught parents of a 20-year-old young man bring him to your office for an evaluation. They state that until recently he had been a model son. In high school, he was active in athletics, had a wide circle of friends, and made good grades. His first semester at college was a disappointment; his grades were mediocre and he seemed withdrawn and distant. They attributed this behavior to his adjustment to living away from home. His second semester was more troubling to his parents. He dropped most of his course work and rarely called or came home. Near the end of the second semester, the parents received a call from a lifelong friend of their son who attends the same college. The friend expressed much concern about the patient, stating that he had ceased attending classes, rarely left his room, and seemed very different from the boy with whom he had grown up. Alarmed, his parents traveled to the college and brought their son home. He has been home for two weeks and they are profoundly worried. The son is markedly withdrawn, refuses to bathe, and is unable to relate to them in any meaningful way. They wondered about substance abuse, but can find no evidence of his using drugs or alcohol. They suspect he is hallucinating and report that he seems to have no energy or interests.

17. Which of the following is/are potential diagnoses?

    1. Schizophrenia
    2. Substance Abuse
    3. Adjustment Disorder
    4. Learning Disorder

18. Which of the following would be reasonable next steps in the management of this patient?

    1. Assess the patient for suicidal/homicidal ideation, explore psychotic symptoms, withhold medications until the diagnosis is clear, and hospitalize only if patient is actively suicidal, homicidal, or grossly out of control.
    2. Hospitalize immediately and begin antipsychotics and drug testing.
    3. Administer psychological tests, obtain academic records, further interview parents, and interview the patient's friend who contacted the parents.
    4. Withhold medication, begin long-term psychotherapy, explore potential parental abuse of patient.

*19–21.* A 45-year-old woman is referred to you by a gynecologist colleague. She states that the patient has never had any medical problems but comes in annually for a PAP smear and a physical examination. The gynecologist was concerned about some of her findings during the last examination of the patient. The patient was noticeably tremulous. Although her sclera and mucous membranes were nonicteric, she had hepatomegaly. The patient reports that she has had a rough year and requests "Valium or something for my nerves." She relates that she and her husband of 20 years are separated and are planning to

divorce. The patient's previously successful business did not do well the past year, and this worries her. The gynecologist is aware that the patient's father and maternal uncle died of alcohol-related complications. The patient readily accepts the psychiatric referral, stating, "I need some help."

19. Which of the following questions might you explore with this patient?

    1. How much alcohol has she been consuming per day?
    2. How much time has elapsed between her last drink and your interview with her?
    3. Does she use any benzodiazepines or other central nervous system (CNS) depressants?
    4. Is there evidence of suicidal ideation and/or impulses?

20. If the patient reported that she was drinking one pint of liquor and consuming 20–40 mg. of diazepam a day, your next step would be to:

    1. Begin an outpatient detoxification schedule.
    2. Refer her to a gastroenterologist.
    3. Maintain her on diazepam but also give disulfiram to enforce abstinence from alcohol.
    4. Hospitalize her in a chemical dependency unit.

21. After the initial phase of detoxification is achieved, which of the following might be useful in helping her maintain sobriety and deal with her life issues?

    1. Psychotherapy
    2. Alcoholics Anonymous (AA)
    3. Education about addictions
    4. Carefully monitored, low-dose benzodiazapines to control her anxiety

*22–23.* A patient positive for the human immunodeficiency virus (HIV) whom you have followed for some time seems to be more confused and cognitively slowed from his baseline function. You are concerned that he is becoming demented.

22. Which of the following symptoms might also be indicative of Dementia Due to HIV Disease?

    1. Balance problems
    2. Fine motor problems
    3. Slowed, dysarthric speech
    4. Aphasia

23. Treatments that might improve the status of the patient include which of the following?

    1. Methylphenidate
    2. Bupropion
    3. Azidothymidine (AZT)
    4. Haloperidol

*24–25.* You are asked to consult on a patient in the intensive care unit. The patient is a 28-year-old African-American man who has developed malignant hypertension. He had not previously been disgnosed with hypertension, and he was rushed to the hospital after having been found comatose by his family. Now he is in full restraints, is unresponsive to verbal stimuli, is highly agitated, and semipurpefully tugs at his intravenous tube. He does not have a nasogastric tube, and he is not intubated. His attending physician is concerned that his agitation and inability to cooperate will compromise his care. Cerebral edema is suspected as the etiology for his delirium. The patient's physician shares with you his concern that the patient may have suffered renal damage and may require dialysis if he survives the acute phase of his illness. Prior to the patient's illness, he was a promising young attorney at a local law firm. He is married to a nurse and they have a 4-year-old son.

24. Which of the following medications would offer both a degree of symptom relief and a margin of safety in the acute control of the patient's delirium?

    1. 250 mg sodium amytal intramuscularly (IM)
    2. 5 mg haloperidol intravenously (IV)
    3. 100 mg chlorpromazine IM
    4. 10 mg diazepam IV

25. Potential long-term issues for this patient might include which of the following?

    1. Sexual dysfunction due to antihypertensive medication
    2. Anger and resentment about the need for dialysis
    3. Regression due to his medical condition
    4. Substance Abuse

26. A middle-aged man brings in his 76-year-old mother for an evaluation. He states that she is "different," although he is unable to describe exactly how she is different. "She's just not herself," he says. The elderly woman is well dressed and groomed and is overtly angry at her son. She adamantly denies that anything is wrong and offers as evidence her continued success in the real estate business that she founded. Indeed, it is well known as a successful and well-run business. The identifed patient's role in the day-to-day operations of the business is confirmed by her partner and employees, yet they also detect that something is "a little off," and they are not sure that the patient is grasping all the details of face-to-face interactions with clients and associates. Her paperwork continues to be of high quality, and she recently purchased and learned to operate a new computer system.Which of the following might be a helpful first step in evaluating this situation?

    1. Neuropsychological testing
    2. Holter monitoring
    3. Urine drug screen
    4. Audiometry

27. You are asked to evaluate a patient's competence for signing an informed consent. Which of the following statements reflect a correct response for a psychiatrist in this situation?

    1. Refer the situation to the hospital attorney since competence is always a legal matter.
    2. Assess the patient's understanding of the disease process, of the treatments available, and of the risks (and potential benefits) of being treated versus not being treated.
    3. 1nform the attending physician that all patients are considered to be competent until deemed incompetent by a judge.
    4. Carefully evaluate and document the patient's mental status.

28–30. A young patient will require long-term maintenance antipsychotic medications to control his Schizophrenia.

28. Which of the following adverse effects will most likely occur during the first 90 days of treatment?

    1. Drug-induced Parkinsonism
    2. Dystonic reactions
    3. Akathisia
    4. Tardive Dyskinesia

29. As a young male, this patient runs the highest risk of which of the following adverse events early in treatment?

    1. Akathisia
    2. Galactorrhea
    3. Parkinsonism
    4. Dystonic reactions

30. In the long-term management of this patient, which of the following would probably enhance the outcome?

    1. Assessing the patient for Tardive Dyskinesia every six months using a standard measurement tool, such as the AIMS
    2. Educating the patient and his family about the nature of his illness, the rationale of the treatment, and any potential adverse effects of the medication
    3. Maintaining a warm and compassionate, but not intrusive, relationship with the patient and his family
    4. Maintaining his antipsychotic medication at a high level to prevent relapse

31–32. Worried family members bring in the 86-year-old matriarch of the family for an evaluation. She is unable to walk, has stopped eating, and today is refusing liquids. Upon being put into bed, she assumes a fetal position, and tightly clutching a rosary, she mumbles about "my sins, my sins." When you ask what the problem is, she replies, "I am so bad... God is punishing me." A thorough medical and neurological exam reveals no acute pathology, except for a mild degree of malnutrition and some dehydration. You decide to transfer her to the psychiatric unit.

31. Which of the following would be a logical next step?

    1. Begin treatment with a selective serotonin reuptake inhibitor.
    2. Insert a nasogastric tube to allow for nutrition, hydration, and medication.

3. Initiate low-dose haloperidol treatment.
4. Plan a course of electroconvulsive therapy (ECT).

32. The patient's family is apprehensive when you suggest ECT, having seen horror stories about the technique in the lay press. Which of the following statements reflect accurate information about ECT?

1. ECT is a very safe treatment for this patient.
2. A prompt response would be expected, usually faster than with oral antidepressants.
3. Depressed elderly persons frequently receive ECT.
4. ECT may interfere with the ability to form new memories after the treatment has been completed.

*33–35.* A 35-year-old woman comes to your office accompanied by her husband. She clings to his arm and wears sunglasses throughout the interview. She is overtly anxious and reports that she can never be alone, rarely leaves her home, is unable to tolerate public places, and cries easily.

33. Which of the following areas should be explored?

1. Her use and/or abuse of substances
2. Depressive symptomatology
3. Symptoms consistent with Panic Attacks
4. Family history of Anxiety Disorders

34. Which of the following medications might be helpful in the management of this patient?

1. Imipramine
2. Fluoxetine
3. Phenelzine
4. Thioridazine

35. In addition to medication, which of the following might be helpful to the patient?

1. Cognitive therapy
2. Relaxation training
3. In vivo exposure
4. Marital therapy

36. A 28-year-old woman comes in for an evaluation. She states that she has a "frog phobia" and wishes to rid herself of this fear of frogs. She says that although she has had a lifelong phobic-level fear of frogs, a recent incident compelled her to seek treatment. Her 4-year-old son fell while playing in the backyard of their suburban home and began crying. As she started out the back door, she abruptly halted, fearing that she would encounter a frog in the yard. A neighbor came to the rescue, and brought the unhurt child inside. The mother states that she feels terrible about the incident and is committed to overcoming her fear of frogs. With regard to the treatment of the patient's Specific Phobia, which of the following statements might be true?

1. Hypnosis is useful in reinforcing the therapist's suggestions that the phobic object is not dangerous.
2. In psychoanalytic treatment settings, the development

of insight generally results in a resolution of the phobia.
3. Desensitization hierarchies may be very useful in the treatment of these phobias.
4. Supportive and family therapy approaches do not have a role in the treatment of these disorders.

*37–38.* You are asked to see a patient who is being treated by a thoracic surgery colleague. The patient is a 59-year-old man who has been hospitalized for the past 10 days for evaluation and irradiation of his esophageal carcinoma. Yesterday, his behavior changed from that of his usual affability. Your exam reveals that he is hyperalert; he picks purposelessly at the bedclothes and seems to be experiencing visual hallucinations. A review of his chart reveals that he has received two to three doses of hydromorphone a day since his admission to the hospital.

37. What is the most likely diagnosis?

1. Brain metastases
2. Dementia due to $B_{12}$ deficiency
3. Alcohol Withdrawal
4. Delirium

38. The drug(s) of choice with which to treat this patient is/are:

1. Chlorpromazine
2. Diazepam
3. Thioridazine
4. Haloperidol

*39–43.* You as the psychiatrist on call are asked to evaluate a newly arrived patient in the emergency room. The patient is a 27-year-old woman who is accompanied by her worried parents and husband. They report she has not slept in four days, seems to be "high" on something, and has been spending money recklessly. She called her elderly grandmother at 3 a.m. the previous morning, greatly upsetting the 83-year-old woman. The patient is an attorney working as an associate in a large law firm and has been described as "brilliant." Her recent behavior is completely uncharacteristic, although she has always been "energetic."

39. Which of the following would contribute to your preliminary diagnosis of Bipolar I Disorder?

1. No family history of Mood Disorder
2. A family history of Substance Abuse, especially alcoholism
3. A history of mood instability in the patient in association with her menstrual cycle
4. No fatigue evident in the patient despite her not sleeping in four days

40. During your interview with the patient, which of the following findings would contribute to a diagnosis of Bipolar I Disorder, Manic Phase?

1. Pressured speech, flight of ideas, agitation

2. Pressured speech, flat affect, grandiose ideation
3. Easy distractibility, bizarre makeup and clothing, lack of judgment
4. Paranoid ideation, loosening of associations, hallucinations

41. Midway through the interview, the patient's mood switches from euphoria to irritability and hostility. Which of the following statements is/are characteristic of this phenomenon?

    1. Is not expected in an untreated manic who has not slept in four days
    2. Usually indicates the patient has been abusing substances
    3. Is not usually due to a failure of interview technique
    4. May indicate that the patient is potentially violent

42. You hospitalize the patient and begin to treat her with lithium carbonate. Which of the following statements about lithium is/are true?

    1. Use in the first trimester of pregnancy may cause a fetal heart malformation.
    2. Nephrogenic diabetes insipidus may result, secondary to, lithium's desensitization of the distal tubules of the kidney to antidiuretic hormone.
    3. It may prevent the release of thyroid hormone from the thyroid gland.
    4. Effect on the cell is mediated by a G-protein receptor that uses cyclic adenosine monophosphate (AMP) as a second messenger.

43. You meet with the family members and try to educate them about the patient's diagnosis. Which of the following is/are correct?

    1. Bipolar Disorder is a genetically transmitted disease involving the incomplete penetrance of an autosomal dominant gene.
    2. Lithium-responsive manic patients have a resolution of their symptoms within seven to 10 days of beginning treatment.
    3. Less time between manic episodes indicates a better long-term prognosis than for patients whose episodes are far apart.
    4. Many manic patients who respond positively to lithium will return to essentially normal functioning.

*44–46.* A 32-year-old woman you have maintained on 40 mg of fluoxetine for several years wants to become pregnant. In the past, she had had severe depressive episodes with active suicidal ideation, but the fluoxetine has brought about a complete and sustained remission of her symptoms. She is employed and is active in her community. Her marital problems related to her depression have abated as a result of the antidepressant treatment and she wants to start a family.

44. Which of the following statements concerning this patient

and her situation is/are true?

    1. The fluoxetine should be slowly tapered and the treating psychiatrist and the obstetrician should collaborate actively in the care of this patient.
    2. This patient is at high risk for postpartum psychiatric problems.
    3. Careful psychiatric monitoring of this patient would be necessary during her pregnancy.
    4. Use of fluoxethine during pregnancy results in a high rate of fetal abnormalities.

45. You decide on a slow taper over two months and see the patient every other week, instructing her to contact you if her depressive symptoms recur. One month into the taper, she announces that she is pregnant. Which of the following might be the next step or steps?

    1. Continue the taper of the fluoxetine
    2. Hospitalize the patient
    3. Stop the fluoxetine
    4. Change to another selective serotonin reuptake inhibitor

46. At four months of gestation, the patient's depressive symptoms have returned to some degree. She is not as depressed as she had been in the past, although both you and the patient know that her current symptoms herald problems to come. Which of the following steps would be resonable to consider taking next?

    1. Instituting a course of ECT
    2. Choosing another antidepressant
    3. Hospitalizing the patient
    4. Restarting the fluoxetine

*47–51.* A longtime patient comes in complaining of increasing difficulties with sleep over the past few months. She is in her late 50s and has always enjoyed good health. She is not on any medication. Two years earlier, her husband of many years died suddenly of a heart attack. You treated her with brief psychotherapy, she did well. Her two grown children are married and live in distant cities. She spontaneously states that she does not feel depressed at the present time, but has trouble going to sleep and staying asleep.

47. In your evaluation of this patient's sleep problem, which of the following would you do?

    1. Ask for more details about symptoms of depression because sleep problems are frequently associated with depression.
    2. Ask about her drinking habits because alcohol can interfere with sleep.
    3. Ask about her use of caffeine-containing food and beverages as caffeine can interfere with sleep.
    4. Refer her to a neurologist because only a sleep laboratory examination can definitively diagnose Sleep Disorders.

48. A review of her medical records reveals that she is three

fourths of an inch shorter than she was ten years earlier. As you prepare to do her physical exam, a hypothesis as to a possible diagnosis forms in your mind. Which of the following physical findings would support your hypothesis?

1. Thinning of scalp hair
2. Evidence of osteoarthritis
3. Thinning and atrophy of vaginal wall
4. Exophthalmus

49. Your evaluation continues with your ordering a complete blood count (CBC), urine analysis, and electrolytes. Among other laboratory tests that might be useful is/are:

1. Rheumatoid factor
2. X-rays of spine and large joints
3. Evaluation of thyroid gland function
4. Plasma estrogen.

50. Two weeks after her initial visit, she returns for your diagnosis and treatment plan. You are almost sure of your diagnosis, and the one question that will clinch the diagnosis is to ask about:

1. Her anxiety about breast cancer
2. Her level of sexual activity
3. Her degree of social isolation and boredom
4. Pain in her joints when at rest, that is less noticeable when she is active

51. Her final diagnosis and its treatment are:

1. Parathyroid gland dysfunction with secondary osteoporosis, osteoarthritis, and pain. Treatment is parathyroid gland replacement, nonsteroidal anti-inflammatory medication, sleeping pills for two weeks.
2. Osteoporosis and osteoarthritis secondary to estrogen deficiency. Treatment is estrogen replacement, narcotic pain relievers, sleep medication for six weeks.
3. Hyperthyroidism with secondary insomnia. Treatment is thyroid surgery, then thyroid gland replacement.
4. Osteoporosis and osteoarthritis secondary to estrogen deficiency. Treatment is estrogen replacement; nonsteroidal, nonnarcotic anti-inflammatory medications indefinitely; sleep medication for two weeks.

# ANSWERS AND EXPLANATIONS

1.  Answer is **d**. Perhaps no condition in child psychiatry presents with such dramatic physical findings. Amenorrhea is present in over 50% of patients before they lose weight, while the remaining patients develop amenorrhea as malnutrition progresses. Among other physical findings are severe weight loss; hypoproteinemia; emaciation with skin pallor, lowered body temperature, pulse rate, and blood pressure, and dryness of the skin and brittleness of the nails; flat or occasionally diabetic blood sugar curves; hypercholesterolemia; hypokalemia secondary to self-induced vomiting and constipation. (*MCCAP 278–279*)

2.  Answer is **a**. Hypothyroidism can result in skin and hair changes, well as amenorrhea. But it always is associated with significant weight gain. Other conditions that may mimic Anorexia Nervosa are pathological lesions of the esophagus, stomach, or duodenum and anterior pituitary insufficiency, or Simmond's disease. (*MCCAP 278–279*)

3.  Answer is **d**. Very often the parents will report that the patient had a history of early feeding problems. Helen may or may not have been obese, but most have only fears or fantasies of becoming fat. Typically what begins as a modest effort to diet quickly turns into an obsessive-compulsive avoidance of food, at times with food binges followed by self-induced vomiting. (*MCCAP 278–279*)

4.  Answer is **e**. Once the condition is diagnosed, treatment should be aggressive and immediate. The patient with Anorexia Nervosa can die of malnutrition. If the patient's body weight is less than 50% of her ideal weight, hospitalization is mandatory. Treatment includes tube feeding or hyperalimentation to provide the necessary calories. Careful weighing of the patient is necessary. (*MCCAP 278–279*)

5.  Answer is **b**. All too often, lip service is paid to the need for close communication. These patients are highly manipulative and will try to interfere with their therapy. (*MCCAP 278–279*)

6.  Answer is **d**. It is rare that the school setting is of any importance for these patients. Often out-of-the-house placement is necessary, as well as public health nurse monitoring. (*MCCAP 278–279*)

7.  Answer is **d**. The most important first step in providing a consultation is to determine what question is being asked, either directly or indirectly, by those requesting the consultation. All of the other steps listed are important to take, but not until you have determined why the consulta-

tion is being requested. (*SP 711–782*)

8.  Answer is **c**. While all of the responses are possibilities to be considered, the most likely explanation for Beth's increased difficulties in controlling her diabetes is that she is struggling with issues of dependence and independence through defensive functions, such as denial, reaction formation and counterphobia. (*SP 711–782*)

9.  Answer **a**. In Prader-Willi syndrome, a genetic disorder, the patient may binge and is very short and grossly overweight. Anorexia Nervosa may seem unlikely because of the patient's weight and the suspicion of self-induced vomiting, but the amount of weight she could have lost is not known at this point and self-induced vomiting has not been established. Bulimia Nervosa seems the most likely diagnosis, but the possibility that the patient vomits as a result of anxiety or other psychogenic causes must be explored. (*MCCAP 278–279*)

10. Answer is **a**. Beth's medical disorder will need continued management. Interrupting her primary relationship with her pediatrician at this point is likely to be harmful for Beth in the long run. Explaining the developmental nature of her disorder must be done in a manner that does not seem condescending to the pediatrician, or this approach could also be damaging. (*SP 711–782*)

11. Answer is **d**. Offering an interpretation before sufficient rapport is established is likely to alienate the nurses, and could increase their anger with you and Beth. (*SP 711–782*)

12. Answer is **c**. There are potential problems with answers b and d, but answer c has the clearest possibility of alienating the family with unsolicited advice, especially before establishing a therapeutic relationship. The family may feel threatened by the request to seek additional information from the family doctor, but this approach may serve as a bridge to help them get into therapy. The direct suggestion that family therapy be utilized may need to be made after another meeting with the family. (*SP 711–782*)

13. Answer is **b**. Although it may be argued that you should notify the authorities immediately, Beth is not in immediate danger and such notification without the involvement of her attending pediatrician may damage your relationship with the with the attending, and subsequently with Beth. It is clear that someone must notify the authorities as soon as possible. It will be up to them to determine the outcome for Beth's family, although you should be available to offer recommendations. (*SP 711–782*)

14. Answer is **e**. As a result of sexual abuse, girls are likely to develop PTSD, Somatization Disorder, Substance abuse, and/or Major Depressive Disorder. Conduct Disorder is also a possibility, but is less likely. Sexually abused boys are likely to develop PTSD, Substance Abuse, and/or Conduct Disorder, and are less likely than are girls to develop Major Depressive Disorder. (*MCCAP 188*)

15. Answer is **c**. While it is desirable that Beth be in favor of the transfer, her agreement is probably the least important of the possibilities listed. The psychiatric unit must agree to manage her diabetes with the consultation of pediatrics. The attending pediatrician must agree that Beth is medically ready to be transferred, and agree to have her followed on the psychiatric unit. If the parents do not cooperate with the transfer to psychiatry, therapy and discharge of Beth become very difficult. (*SP 711–782*)

16. Answer is **e**. In the long run, however, answers c and d should prove to be the most likely. Based on the limited amount of information available regarding Beth's coping abilities and early life experiences, it is probably too early to say for certain what Beth's prognosis will be. However, based on the probabilities of the outcomes of Bulimia Nervosa and sexual abuse, Beth's prognosis is fair at best, and may be poor. (*MCCAP 284*)

17. Answer is **A**. The patient does not have historical evidence of a learning problem given his good academic record in high school. The psychotic symptomatology described might support a diagnosis of Schizophrenia, as would his impaired relatedness skills and isolation. He could be experiencing an Adjustment Disorder since he has been away from home for the first time and could be undergoing difficulties owing to his new environment and circumstances. He could also be using and/or abusing substances. His college environment may have exposed him to drugs and his use of these substances could have produced his behavior and symptoms. (*SP 475–480*)

18. Answer is **A**. While a case could be made for all of the steps suggested, the next step should focus on gathering information to clarify symptoms and develop a diagnosis. This process could be accomplished on an outpatient basis if the patient is not homicidal, suicidal, or out of control. His parents seem supportive and caring. Other sources of information, such as academic records, his friend, and psychological testing, would help to flesh out the picture of this patient. Maintaining a good rapport with the patient through all this would be difficult but essential. Abruptly hospitalizing and medicating the patient without a firm diagnosis might do more harm than good, but may be necessary. Initiating a treatment, such as a psychotherapeutic process, would be premature at this juncture. In addition, entering an exploratory process with a preconceived notion, such as of parental abuse, will contaminate both the data needed for diagnosis and the relationship needed for treatment. (*SP 481–485*)

19. Answer is **E**. The patient's drug and alcohol use certainly need to be explored, as well as the details of such use. Alcohol consumed in combination with benzodiazepines or other CNS depressants can be fatal. Asking how much time has elapsed since her last drink is important since alcohol withdrawal begins within 12 hours (and often in less time) after the last drink. Also, whether the patient appears to be intoxicated or in withdrawal during the interview would be important to note. A direct and complete exploration of any suicidal ideation or impulses would be an essential part of the interview. (*SP 396–406*)

20. Answer is **D**. This patient has a serious Substance Abuse problem that will require the support and care available only on an inpatient unit, preferably a chemical dependency unit. The possibility that she will be able to remain abstinent from alcohol even with disulfiram is remote and potentially dangerous due to side effects from drinking while taking disulfiram. For the same reasons, the likelihood of success with an outpatient detox program is slight. Her coming to the appointment is a clear indication of her desire for help, and it may indicate that she feels out of control. Once she is hospitalized, a gastroenterologist can be consulted to evaluate the hepatic and gastrointestinal sequelae of her alcohol abuse. (*SP 409–410*)

21. Answer is **A**. Psychotherapy together with active participation in AA and education about the disease process of addiction are a potent combination for many who are entering a recovery process. Use of potentially addicting CNS depressants such as benzodiazepines, runs the risk of reigniting the use/abuse cycle and aborting attempts to learn new ways to deal with stress and anxiety. (*SP 408–410*)

22. Answer is **A**. Dementia Due to HIV Disease is a subcortical dementia characterized by dysarthric speech, motor problems, and balance problems. Patients also complain of poor concentration and a dulling of their cognitive capacities. Fine motor skills, such as handwriting, may be affected. Aphasia is characteristic of cortical dementia, such as Dementia of the Alzheimer's Type, and is not a feature of Dementia Due to HIV Disease. Insight is preserved well into the dementing process in the latter type of dementia, tending to be lost earlier in the course of the cortical dementias. (*SP 378–781*)

23. Answer is **A**. Patients with HIV may benefit from high-dose AZT earlier in their dementing process, although many cannot tolerate the doses required for penetration into the brain. Medications that enhance dopaminergic transmission seem to have a positive effect on the symptoms, especially the cognitive symptoms. Methylphenidate (Ritalin) and bupropion (Wellbutrin) have been used to improve the symptoms of such patients.

Haloperidol and other dopamine receptor antagonists should be avoided as these medications may make the cognitive and motor problems worse. (*SP 381–382*)

24. Answer is **C**. In a nonintubated patient with cerebral and potential respiratory and cardiovascular problems, neither barbiturates nor low-potency phenothiazine should be used. Barbiturates may cause respiratory arrest and marked hypotension can occur with the use of low-potency agents, especially via the IM route. Although IV haloperidol is quite safe, it is underutilized in the United States. It has no associated cardiac or respiratory effects, and side effects, such as Acute Dystonia, are lowest with the IV route. Intravenous diazepam has long been used to premedicate patients for procedures and is relatively safe. Older patients, however, may be sensitive to the respiratory suppressant effects of diazepam and require careful observation. The gamma-aminobutyric acid (GABA) receptor antagonist flumazenil also makes this a safe choice since it will reverse any adverse effects. (*SP 344*)

25. Answer is **A**. The sudden onset of severe medical illness is always a tremendous stress, especially in the young and if the disease process requires intrusive and continuous treatment procedures. With all patients on antihypertensives, sexual dysfunction can be a major problem and should be addressed to help the patient maintain compliance. Patients requiring intrusive, time-consuming, and repetitive medical procedures are often angry and resentful about their situation. Regression resulting from many factors, such as dependence on technology to live and family members' reactions to the illness, is often seen in these circumstances. Having a health care professional as a spouse may be either a boon or a problem, depending on the spouse's reaction to the medical situation. If Substance Abuse was not a problem prior to the illness, it probably will not become a new problem. Patients with a strong genetic predisposition for addiction problems might bear careful watching. Helping a patient in these circumstances to develop good coping strategies is the best way to prevent such reactions as becoming depressed or abusing alcohol or drugs. (*SP 775–782*)

26. Answer is **D**. In the older person, hearing deficits are frequently overlooked as a possible source of problems in dealing with the environment, especially in interacting with others. This hypothetical patient's performance in the cognitive area is unimpaired, and indeed she is able to learn new skills. The inability to acquire new knowledge and skills is one of the hallmarks of dementia. Substance Abuse by elderly persons also is frequently overlooked; such abuse most often involves prescription medications and/or alcohol. But our patient's work performance and appearance belie this diagnosis. Neurological evaluation and Holter monitoring are useful tools but possibly not as a first step. Careful attention to the patient's responses to

verbal stimuli and a referral for an audiometric evaluation might clarify the situation. (*SP 296–297, 351–355*)

27. Answer is **E**. The question of competence is a complex one, but it is basically a legal issue. This does not allow physicians to ignore it, however. For the sake of both doctor and patient, the issue merits careful attention. In the United States, all citizens are deemed competent to handle their own affairs unless a court decides they are incompetent. Courts are usually reluctant to abridge the civil rights of a patient, and this may produce a difficult clinical situation. The psychiatrist can contribute by clarifying the patient's mental status in detail and evaluating the three general areas of competence: the patient's understanding of the disease process, of the treatments available, and of the risks and potential benefits of allowing the treatment to proceed or of choosing not to be treated. No physician (including a psychiatrist) may determine the competency of a patient, unless the doctor is also a judge. (*SP 1178-1180*)

28. Answer is **A**. As its name implies, Tardive Dyskinesia is a late-occurring event, usually after at least 6 months of treatment. Dystonic reactions, drug-induced parkinsonism, and akathisia are all early events in the course of treatment. (*SP 949–953*)

29. Answer is **D**. Dystonic reactions are particularly likely to occur in young males early in the course of treatment. All of the other adverse events—bradykinesia, galactorrhea, akathisia, and parkinsonism—may also arise during the course of treatment. (*SP 947–951*)

30. Answer is **A**. The dose of the antipsychotic should be the lowest that will keep his symptoms at bay. The patient should be assessed with a standard measure to determine the presence of any Tardive Dyskinesia. This information should be entered into the patient's medical record. Appropriate education of the patient and his family would greatly increase the likelihood of compliance and avoid adverse medication effects. Use of medications to diminish or prevent side effects should also be part of the treatment plan. An appropriately warm, supportive and compassionate professional relationship can be invaluable in helping the patient to achieve a measure of stability. (*SP 481–485*)

31. Answer is **D**. The patient is most likely psychotically depressed and may respond best, and most rapidly, to a course of ECT. Since she is refusing oral intake, attempting to begin an oral regimen would be futile. The insertion of the nasogastric tube may be fraught with problems. Antidepressants take three to six weeks for their effects to be realized, and in that time the patient could develop decubitus ulcers, aspiration pneumonia, esophageal erosion from the nasogastric tube, or a host of other avoidable problems. (*SP 1155–1165*)

**32.** Answer is **A**. ECT may cause the permanent loss of memories of the events that led up to the hsopitalization and of parts of the hospitalization itself, but most patients recover full memory function within six months after treatment. The patients who respond most poorly to the antidepressant effects of ECT seem to have the greatest memory problems. The depressed elderly are often the group most frequently treated with ECT. It causes a prompt antidepressant effect, often more quickly than do oral antidepressants. In this group of patients, ECT is very safe. Some patients benefit from maintenance ECT. (*SP 1005–1010*)

**33.** Answer is **E**. All of these areas should be explored in assessing this patient. Her complaints are consistent with Agoraphobia, but Agoraphobia is not a codable diagnosis in DSM-IV. With regard to her possible use of alcohol, sedative-hypnotics may be utilized in an attempt to control her symptoms, or they may contribute to the production of symptoms. Depressive syndromes could also play a role in the genesis of this patient's problems. Panic Disorder With Agoraphobia would be high on the list of possible diagnoses, and any symptoms associated with Panic Attacks should be investigated. Anxiety Disorders tend to "run" in families, and the type, and any treatment, of Anxiety Disorders in family members should be documented. (*SP 585–589*)

**34.** Answer is **A**. Imipramine has long been used to treat anxiety and depression. It is especially helpful in the treatment of Panic Disorder. Newer antidepressants, such as fluoxetine, sertraline, and paroxetine, have also proved useful in the treatment of anxious patients. The monamine oxidase inhibitors, such as phenelzine, are helpful in the management of these disorders, as well. The antipsychotics, such as thioridazine, do not have a role in the treatment of such disorders. (*SP 589–590*)

**35.** Answer is **E**. All of these therapeutic approaches may prove to be helpful to the patient. Cognitive and behavioral techniques are very useful in the treatment of these disorders. In vivo exposure may be used to help the patient overcome anxiety about specific activities or settings, such as grocery shopping. If the Agoraphobia has continued for any length of time, marital or family therapy may be indicated to address the disruption caused by the disorder. (*SP 590–591*)

**36.** Answer is **B**. Early in the development of psychoanalysis, Freud and others realized that, in treating these disorders, the therapist should urge the patient to seek out the phobic object and to experience both the anxiety and the insight in order to improve. Merely gaining insight is not enough. Hypnosis may be very helpful in reinforcing the therapist's suggestions that the phobic object is not dangerous. Desensitization techniques, as pioneered by Wolpe, have proved to be very valuable in treating such disorders. Family therapy may be of use in supporting the family and the patient as the treatment proceeds. Supportive techniques may help as well. (*SP 597*)

**37.** Answer is **D**. This patient is delirious. Brain metastases might be a possibility but could easily be ruled out and would not likely be part of this clinical picture. A deficiency of $B_{12}$ (nicotinamide) results in memory disturbances, confusion, depression, insomnia, and psychosis, but this, too, is unlikely in this patient. The patient's symptoms began too long after his admission to the hospital to be attributable to Alcohol Withdrawal, and with proper shielding and beam focus, radiation exposure as a cause would be unlikely. The most likely cause is the hydromorphone (Dilaudid) that the patient is receiving. Narcotic analgesics are common causes of delirium in hospitalized patients. (*SP 338–343, 774*)

**38.** Answer is **D**. Haloperidol is the drug of choice in the treatment of a delirium. The suspected offending agent should be removed, and usually low-dose haloperidol will greatly assist in the patient's recovery. Low-potency antipsychotics, such as chlorpromazine and thioridazine, would not be useful because at their high anticholinergic activity and their potential for worsening the delirium. Anxiolytics would have little place in the treatment of this condition. (*SP 344*)

**39–43.** Answers are: 39, **C**; 40, **B**; 41, **B**; 42, **A**; 43, **C**. Family history of alcoholism and Mood Disorder is a common finding in patients with Bipolar Disorder. A lack of fatigue in spite of loss of sleep is a hallmark symptom of mania. Mood instability in association with the menstrual cycle is not associated with Bipolar Disorder.

Manic patients exhibit all of the characteristics listed in all of the selections in question 40, except flat affect. Usually the manic patient will have an exaggerated affective display.

Untreated manic patients will often develop irritablity as the illness continues. The switch would not be unexpected in this patient and most likely would not be due to substance abuse or a failure of the interviewing technique. Irritable manic patients can suddenly become violent and assaultive and should be carefully watched for this development.

As the episode resolves with treatment, the irritability will abate. Lithium's effects are mediated by G-protein receptors, but seem to be linked to the phosphatidylinositol second-messenger systems. Its use during pregnancy may result in a fatal heart malformation in the developing fetus (Ebstein's malformation), and while the incidence of this defect is low (3%), its nearly always fatal outcome warrants the determination of the pregnancy status of a patient before beginning treatment.

Polyuria due to the desensitization of the distal renal tubules to the actions of antidiuretic hormone is a well-known effect of lithium administration. Equally well known is lithium's effects on the thyroid gland, with the blockade of the release of thyroid hormones becoming a significant problem in some patients. About 50% of all lithium-treated patients develop a fine motor tremor that may reduce compliance if not treated. Low-dose propranolol will relieve the tremor in most patients. (*SP 532–535, 961–969*)

44. Answer is **A**. Fluoxetine is not associated with fetal abnormalities when taken during pregnancy. Abnormalities seen in infants exposed to fluoxetine in utero do not differ in type or number from those in the general population. This patient is at high risk for postpartum psychiatric problems, especially postpartum depression. Careful monitoring throughout her pregnancy for the emergence of depressive symptoms would be essential, as would an active collaboration with her obstetrician. A slow taper of the fluoxetine while maintaining birth control would be a prudent course for this patient. (*SP 976–980*)

45. Answer is **B**. With the very low risk to the fetus that continuing the taper poses, this could be a reasonable choice. Discontinuing the medication would also be a reasonable choice. The patient does not require hospitalization at the present time and switching to another selective serotonin reuptake inhibitor would not be a logical step. (*SP 976–980*)

46. Answer is **D**. With its documented safety in pregnancy and this patient's history of positive response, fluoxetine would be the treatment of choice. Her potential response to ECT or to other medications is unknown. Her symptoms are not of a magnitude to require her hospitalization. (*SP 872, 976–980*)

*47–51.* Answers are: 47, **D**; 48, **A**; 49, **C**; 50, **D**; 51, **D**. This seemingly complex situation is actually common and simple. This patient has osteoarthritis and osteoporosis, both of which are producing chronic low-grade pain that is hardly noticeable during a busy day, but is quite significant at night when the level of stimulation, and hence distraction, drops. The patient is uncomfortable and unable to fall asleep. Pain is a very common cause of insomnia that is frequently overlooked. Depression could also be a cause, especially in this previously depressed patient. However, having undergone psychotherapy with you in the past, she would probably be forthcoming about any depressive symptoms. (*SP 704*)

# 6

# PRACTICE
# EXAMINATION

# QUESTIONS

**DIRECTIONS: For the following questions, select the single best answer.**

1. All of the following are true of Tardive Dyskinesia **EXCEPT**:
   a. It occurs shortly after initiation of treatment.
   b. It is absent during sleep.
   c. It may be treatment resistant.
   d. It is a movement disorder.
   e. It is related to the use of antipsychotic medications.

2. Which of the following statements is true?
   a. A positive dexamethasone-suppression test (DST) indicates the possible presence of depression.
   b. The normalization of the DST is an indication that it is safe to discontinue antidepressants.
   c. False positive and false negative results are rare with this test.
   d. The sensitivity of the DST for Major Depressive Disorder is 90%.

3. Which of the following statements about the neurological adverse effects of the dopamine receptor antagonists is false?
   a. Men are twice as frequently affected by Neuroleptic-Induced Parkinsonism than are women.
   b. Akathisia usually occurs within the first 90 days of the onset of treatment.
   c. Tardive Dyskinesia rarely occurs until after six months of treatment.
   d. Tardive Dyskinesia may remit spontaneously in mild cases.
   e. With depot antipsychotic medications, the mortality may reach 20–30% if the patient develops the Neuroleptic Malignant Syndrome.

4. Which of the following can result from the use of lithium by pregnant women?
   a. Ebstein's malformation, an anomaly of the bicuspid valve, that commonly occurs in fetuses exposed to lithium in the first trimester of pregnancy, has a low morbidity and mortality rate.
   b. Ebstein's malformation rarely occurs in fetuses exposed to lithium in the first trimester of pregnancy, but has a high mortality rate.
   c. Esophageal atresia
   d. Spina bifida
   e. Craniofacial abnormalities

5. Which of the following statements is not true?
   a. Lithium may cause benign leukocytosis.
   b. Thrombocytopenia may be a problem with carbamazepine.

   c. Monoamine oxidase inhibitors and selective serotonin reuptake inhibitors are a common and safe combination for treatment-resistant depression.
   d. Venlafaxine should be avoided in hypertensive patients.
   e. Lithium and antidepressants are a common and safe combination in the treatment of Bipolar I Disorder.

6. High-potency antipsychotic medications:
   a. Most often cause acute dystonic reactions in elderly women.
   b. Are quite anticholinergic.
   c. May result in bradykinesia.
   d. Should not be used in patients with history of cardiac problems.
   e. Should always be given in high doses to achieve maximum therapeutic effect.

7. Characteristics of a patient during a Manic Episode include all of the following **EXCEPT**:
   a. Manic patients are talkative, excited, and hyperactive.
   b. About 75% of all manic patients are delusional, assaultive, and threatening.
   c. Impaired judgment is a hallmark of mania.
   d. Early in the course of mania, patients are most often irritable, becoming more euphoric as the episode progresses.
   e. In acute mania, speech may be completely incoherent and indistinguishable from that of a patient with Schizophrenia.

8. All of the following statements regarding Major Depressive Disorder are true **EXCEPT**:
   a. Decreased rate and volume of speech are common in depressed patients.
   b. Not all depressed patients may appear to be depressed and may deny depressive symptoms.
   c. Hallucinations and other perceptual problems occur in most depressed patients.
   d. Impaired attention and concentration are common in depressed patients.
   e. Disorientation is not common in depressed patients.

9. Which of the following statements is true?
   a. All known antipsychotic medications that are effective have an affinity for the $D_2$ receptor.
   b. Dystonic reactions to these drugs are most common in middle-aged women.
   c. In schizophrenic patients, the antipsychotic medications work best in the alleviation of the positive symptoms of Schizophrenia.
   d. Antipsychotic medications are effective only in treating psychotic symptoms due to Schizophrenia.

e. High-potency antipsychotic medications are more cardiotoxic than are low-potency agents.

10. Bipolar I Disorder:

a. Refers to a clinical situation in which the patient experiences a period of Hypomania followed by a Major Depressive Disorder.

b. Refers to a clinical situation in which the patient exhibits a complete set of symptoms for mania over the course of the illness.

c. Refers to a clinical situation in which the mania is clearly caused by an external agent, such as an antidepressant.

d. Cannot be referred to as having a Rapid-Cycling subtype.

11. The DSM-IV criteria for the diagnosis of a Major Depressive Episode include all of the following EXCEPT:

a. Insomnia or hypersomnia nearly every day

b. Significant weight change without the patient's trying to gain or lose weight

c. Recurrent thoughts of death or suicide

d. Symptoms present nearly every day for a month

e. Depressed mood most of the day nearly every day or loss of interest or pleasure

12. All of the following are appropriate actions to take when dealing with a violent patient EXCEPT:

a. Have adequate personnel available for the management of the patient before interviewing the patient.

b. Ignore any gut feeling about the potential dangerousness of the patient.

c. Carefully observe violent patients who have been sedated with medications.

d. Warn individuals against whom the patient expresses specific threats.

e. Do not bargain with violent patients.

13. Regarding the etiology of Schizophrenia, which of the following is true?

a. Cerebrospinal fluid levels of homovanillic acid are abnormally low in patients with Schizophrenia.

b. The tuberoinfundibular tract has been implicated in the pathogenesis of Schizophrenia.

c. Schizophrenic patients may show enlargement of the third and lateral ventricles of the brain on computerized tomography (CT).

d. Serotonin and norepinephrine do not play a role in the development of Schizophrenia.

e. The dopamine 4 receptor (D4) plays the key role in the pathogenesis of Schizophrenia.

14. A 30-year-old woman, who is being treated for depression, while attending a party begins to complain of a severe headache. She is taken to a local emergency room, where physical examination reveals a blood pressure of 230/135 mm Hg, dilated pupils, and diaphoresis. She

reports that she had eaten cheese and chicken liver pâté. This woman probably has been taking:

a. Lithium carbonate

b. A tricyclic antidepressant

c. A monoamine oxidase inhibitor

d. A phenothiazine

e. A butyrophenone

15. The Neuroleptic Malignant Syndrome is characterized by all of the following EXCEPT:

a. Hyperthermia

b. Muscle rigidity

c. Hypertension

d. Confusion

e. Paranoia

16. In the treatment of an acute Manic Episode, the blood level of lithium should be:

a. 0.1 to 0.2 mEq/L

b. 0.2 to 0.5 mEq/L

c. 0.8 to 1.2 mEqL

d. 1.2 to 2.4 mEq/L

e. 2.4 to 3.0 mEq/L

17. Tricyclic antidepressant medications can cause all of the following EXCEPT:

a. Widening of the QRS interval

b. Depressed ST segments

c. Atrial fibrillation

d. Flattening of T waves

e. Tachycardia

18. What proportion of patients with Schizophrenia eventually commit suicide?

a. About 1 %

b. About 3%

c. About 5%

d. About 10%

e. About 50%

19. Compared with suicide attempters, suicide completers are more likely to be:

a. Younger

b. Male

c. Impulsive in planning the attempt

d. Acting when help is available

e. Suffering from a Personality Disorder

20. Which of the following is associated with a particularly poor prognosis for Schizophrenia?

a. Acute onset

b. Affective symptoms

c. Clouded sensorium

d. Positive family history of Schizophrenia

e. Marriage

21. All of the following statements about akathisia are correct EXCEPT:

a. Motor restlessness may be confused with agitation.
b. It is not caused by inner anxiety.
c. Propranolol may produce symptomatic relief.
d. It is improved by increasing antipsychotic dose.
e. Amantadine often is therapeutic.

22. Early manifestations of lithium toxicity include all of the following **EXCEPT**:

   a. Convulsions
   b. Ataxia
   c. Lethargy
   d. Nystagmus
   e. Vomiting

23. The most dangerous symptom resulting from tricyclic antidepressant overdose is:

   a. Coma
   b. Recurrent seizures
   c. Renal failure
   d. Cardiac arrhythmias
   e. Hallucinations

24. An increased risk of suicide among the elderly is associated with all of the following **EXCEPT**:

   a. Divorce
   b. Alcoholism
   c. Male gender
   d. Chronic illness
   e. Belonging to a minority group

25. When Bipolar Disorder is designated Type ll, this indicates:

   a. Major Depressive and Manic Episodes
   b. Major Depressive and Hypomanic Episodes
   c. Dysthymic Disorder and Manic Episodes
   d. Major Depressive Disorder superimposed on Dysthymic Disorder
   e. Major Depressive Disorder with Melancholia

26. Hypnagogic hallucinations are:

   a. False perceptions of insects crawling on the skin
   b. False perceptions when falling asleep
   c. Sensations perceived in a different sensory modality
   d. False perceptions associated with alcohol abuse
   e. Misperceptions about real external stimuli

27. Which of the following life events has been rated as causing the greatest degree of stress?

   a. Divorce
   b. Death of spouse
   c. Jail term
   d. Marital separation
   e. Death of a sibling

28. Physiological symptoms of stress may include all of the following **EXCEPT**:

   a. Muscle tension
   b. Headaches

c. Bradycardia
d. Anorexia Nervosa
e. Insomnia

29. The literature concerning the problem of patient noncompliance indicates all of the following **EXCEPT**:

   a. The rate of noncompliance or nonadherence to treatment plans may vary between 20% and 80%.
   b. The seriousness of a disease and the amount of technical knowledge the patient has about the illness increase compliance and adherence.
   c. Patient compliance tends to be promoted by the presence of a continuous, warm, and positive patient–practitioner relationship.
   d. Demographic variables, a patient's personality, characteristics of the patient, and clinical judgment among experienced practitioners are not reliable predictors of patient compliance.
   e. Expensive therapy, prolonged waiting hours, and lack of continuity of care encourage noncompliance.

30. Of the following, the least common manifestation of a Depressive Disorder in an elderly person is:

   a. Loss of appetite
   b. Significant weight loss
   c. Severe fatigue
   d. Absence of somatic complaints
   e. Sleeplessness

31. The correct order of antipsychotics according to potency, high to low, is:

   a. Thiothixene, haloperidol, chlorpromazine
   b. Haloperidol, chlorpromazine, thiothixene
   c. Chlorpromazine, thiothixene, haloperidol
   d. Haloperidol, thiothixene, chlorpromazine
   e. Chlorpromazine, haloperidol, thiothixene

32. Patient compliance with psychotropic medication can be increased by all of the following **EXCEPT**:

   a. Making sure that the purpose of the medication is clear to the patient.
   b. Dividing up the daily dosage so the patient does not have to take too many pills at once.
   c. Rapidly treating side effects.
   d. Involving patients, as much as possible, in their own medication management.
   e. Making sure medication instructions are understood.

33. Indicate whether the adverse effects would be high (a), medium (b), or low (c).

| | Sedation | Anticholinergic | Hypotension | Extrapyramidal |
|---|---|---|---|---|
| Chloropromazine | (1) | (2) | (3) | (4) |
| Haloperidol | (5) | (6) | (7) | (8) |
| Loxapine | (9) | (10) | (11) | (12) |
| Molindone | (13) | (14) | (15) | (16) |
| Trifluoperazine | (17) | (18) | (19) | (20) |

**DIRECTIONS: For questions 34–53, select:**

  **A.** If the item is associated with **a** only
  **B.** If the item is associated with **b** only
  **C.** If the item is associated with both **a** and **b**
  **D.** If the item is associated with neither **a** nor **b**

    **a.** Tricyclic antidepressants
    **b.** Selective serotonin reuptake inhibitors
    **c.** Both
    **d.** Neither

34. Dopaminergic

35. Block reuptake of serotonin

36. alpha-adenergic blockade

37. Block reuptake of norepinephrine

38. Block action of monoamine oxidase

39. Orthostatic hypotension

40. Nausea

41. Weight gain

42. Somnulence

43. Priapism

44. Concurrent use with monamine oxidase inhibitors is an absolute contraindication.

45. Cardiac arrhythmia in overdose situation

46. Three-week onset of action

47. Block action of cytochrome P450 system

48. Usually given in a single morning dose

49. Urinary retention

50. Sexual dysfunction

51. Blurred vision

52. Insomnia

53. Movement disorders

**DIRECTIONS: For questions 54–63, select:**

  **A.** If the item is associated with **a** only
  **B.** If the item is associated with **b** only
  **C.** If the item is associated with both **a** and **b**
  **D.** If the item is associated with neither **a** nor **b**

    **a.** Dementia
    **b.** Delirium
    **c.** Both
    **d.** Neither

54. Reduced level of consciousness

55. Memory impairment

56. Fluctuating course over span of a day

57. Most often, slow onset of months to years

58. Hallucinations may occur

59. Memory impairment a prominent feature

60. Unimpaired level of alertness

61. Treating underlying cause results in prompt improvement.

62. "Personality change"

63. Widespread cortical dysfunction

**DIRECTIONS: Questions 64–73 list diagnostic criteria for Panic Disorder and Generalized Anxiety Disorder. Match each criterion to the appropriate disorder:**

    **a.** Panic Disorder
    **b.** Generalized Anxiety Disorder
    **c.** Both
    **d.** Neither

64. Shortness of breath

65. Fear of dying

66. Exaggerated startle response

67. Decreased energy

68. Dizziness

69. Derealization or depersonalization

70. Nausea

71. Difficulty concentrating

72. Trembling or shaking

73. Fear of going crazy

**Match each adverse effect with the correct clinical result listed in questions 74–83.**

    a. Antidopaminergic adverse effect
    b. Antiadrenergeric adverse effect
    c. Antihistaminergic adverse effect

74. Dizziness

75. Menstrual dysfunction

76. Weight gain

77. Sedation

78. Sexual dysfunction

79. Parkinsonism

80. Reflex tachycardia

81. Hyperprolactinemia

82. Akathisia

83. Tardive dyskinesia

**Match the elements of the mental status exam with the clinical findings listed in questions 84–108.**

    a. Appearance
    b. Behavior
    c. Attitude toward examiner
    d. Affect
    e. Speech
    f. Perceptual disturbance
    g. Thought process
    h. Thought content
    i. Orientation
    j. Insight
    k. Mood

84. Loosening of associations

85. Hallucinations

86. Awareness that one is ill

87. Delusions

88. Hostility

89. Circumstantial

90. Disheveled

91. Outward expression of emotion

92. Date

93. Subjective feeling state

94. Loudness

95. Derealization

96. Groomlng

97. Logical

98. Place

99. Seductive

100. Agitation

101. Digit span

102. Formication

103. Preoccupation

104. Monotone

105. Inappropriate to thought content

106. Awareness of need for treatment

107. Awareness of location and situation

108. Echopraxia

**For questions 109–113, indicate which of the following applies.**

    a. Both fact and reason are true
    b. Fact is false, but reason is true
    c. Fact is true, but reason is false
    d. Both fact and reason are false

109. Frequent complete blood counts (CBCs) are required when treating a patient with Clozaril because Clozaril can cause decreased white blood cell counts.

110. Negative symptoms of Schizophrenia respond most favorably to antipsychotic medication because antipsychotic medications block $D_2$ dopamine receptors.

111. Patients with Paranoid Type Schizophrenia have severe loosening of associations because the disorder involves systematized delusions.

112. Hospitalization of patients with Schizophrenia decreases their level of stress because hospitalization provides a safe, stable, supportive environment.

113. Patients with Scizophrenia may respond well to dopaminergic antagonists because only schizophrenics have the disordered cerebral neurochemistry that respond to the dopaminergic antagonists.

114. All of the following medications have proven effective in the treatment of Panic Disorder **EXCEPT**:

    a. Imipramine
    b. Thioridazine
    c. Phenelzine
    d. Alprazolam
    e. Fluoxetine

115. All of the following are true about lithium carbonate **EXCEPT**:

    a. It is a cheap, easily produced inorganic salt.
    b. It achieves complex steady-state equilibrium in 10–12 days.
    c. Its excretion is unaffected by hydrochlorothiazide.
    d. Its excretion is unaffected by furosemide.
    e. Cerebrospinal fluid (CSF) levels are 50% of peripheral blood levels after equilibrium has been achieved.

116. All of the following statements about patients with Panic Disorder are true **EXCEPT**:

    a. They may initially attempt to keep their symptoms a secret.
    b. They should reduce caffeine intake.
    c. Approximately 50% will have a spontaneous remission if followed long term.
    d. They frequently are also depressed
    e. They have a 50% chance of having comorbid Substance Abuse Disorder

117. All of the following statements about the locus ceruleus are correct **EXCEPT**:

    a. It contains most of the cell bodies for most of the noradrenergic neurons in the brain.
    b. It is located in caudal pons.
    c. Its neurons project to limbic system, brain stem, and spinal cord.
    d. Ablation in monkeys decreases fear response.
    e. It receives sensory input regarding pain

**Match the type of Schizophrenia with the items listed in questions 118–127.**

    a. Disorganized Type of Schizophrenia
    b. Catatonic Type of Schizophrenia
    c. Paranoid Type of Schizophrenia

118. Late onset

119. Marked regression to primitive unorganized behavior

120. May rapidly alternate between stupor and excitement

121. Rare in Europe and North America

122. Thought disorder most pronounced

123. Delusions predominate

124. Intelligence preserved

125. Frequent outbursts of inappropriate laughter

126. Ideas of reference

127. Waxy flexibility

**Match the prevalence rate with the items listed in questions 128–133.**

    a. 1.0% prevalence of Schizophrenia
    b. 8.0% prevalence of Schizophrenia
    c. 12.0% prevalence of Schizophrenia
    d. 40% prevalence of Schizophrenia
    e. 47% prevalence of Schizophrenia

128. Dizygotic twin of schizophrenic patient

129. General population

130. Child of two schizophrenic parents

131. Child with one schizophrenic parent

132. Nontwin sibling of a schizophrenic patient

133. Monozygotic twin of schizophrenic patient

# ANSWERS AND EXPLANATIONS

1. **Answer is a.** Tardive Dyskinesia develops after six months of treatment. It completely disappears during sleep and may be quite treatment resistant, although mild cases may remit spontaneously. By definition, it is a movement disorder related to the use of dopamine receptor antagonists. (*SP 951–952*)

2. **Answer is a.** The DST may help confirm a clinical impression of depression but only 45% of patients with a diagnosis of Major Depressive Disorder will have a positive DST. Normalization of the DST is not an indication to stop treatment, and false positives and negatives are common. (*SP 283*)

3. **Answer is a.** Women are twice as frequently affected by Neuroleptic Induced Parkinsonism as are men. Both parkinsonism and akathisia occur early in the course of treatment. Tardive Dyskinesia develops after six months of treatment, and mild cases may spontaneously remit. The mortality rate for the Neuroleptic Malignant Syndrome in patients treated with depot medications may be as high as 20–30%. (*SP 949–953*)

4. **Answer is b.** The Ebstein's malformation occurs in about 3% of fetuses exposed to lithium in the first trimester of pregnancy. Although rare, it is usually fatal, and thus pregnant women should not receive lithium. Esophageal atresia, spina bifida, and craniofacial abnormalities are not associated with lithium use in pregnancy. (*SP 966*)

5. **Answer is c.** Monoamine oxidase inhibitors and selective serotonin reuptake inhibitors cannot be used together. A hyyperserotoninergic syndrome results, with a high mortality rate. Lithium may cause a significant, although benign, leukocytosis and thrombocytopenia may result with carbamazepine. In high doses, venlafaxine may accelerate hypertension. Lithium combines well with antidepressants in the treatment of Bipolar I Disorder. (*SP 926, 963, 964, 979 1003*)

6. **Answer is c.** High-potency antipsychotics may result in significant bradykinesia. Acute dystonic reactions are most common in young males. These agents have low anticholinergic activity and are safe in cardiac patients. The lowest possible dose to maintain symptom remission should be used in order to minimize adverse effects. (*SP 947, 948, 950*)

7. **Answer is d.** Early in mania, patients are euphoric, but if the episode progresses unchecked, the patient will become more irritable. The manic patient is loquacious, excited, and hyperactive. Seventy-five percent of such patients will be delusional, assaultive, or threatening. During acute mania, the speech may become so incoherent as to resemble that of a patient experiencing an acute schizophrenic episode. (*SP 532*)

8. **Answer is c.** Most patients with Depressive Disorder do not experience hallucinations or other perceptual problems, although such problems may be severe in some patients. Disorientation is not common in depressed patients, but decreased rate and volume of speech, as well as impaired attention and concentration, are common symptoms. (*SP 523–525*)

9. **Answer is c.** Positive symptoms, such as hallucinations and delusions, respond best to these medications. Psychotic symptoms of any origin will respond to the medications as well. The new antipsychotic medication clozapine does not have a high affinity for $D_2$ receptors and is an effective antipsychotic. Young males most frequently experience dystonic reactions to these drugs. The low-potency antipsychotics are much more cardiotoxic than are the high-potency agents (*SP 944–947*)

10. **Answer is b.** Bipolar I Disorder refers to a clinical syndrome characterized by full-blown mania alternating with Major Depressive Episodes. Bipolar II Disorder is a period of Hypomania preceding a Major Depressive Episode. Rapid-Cycling Bipolar I Disorder is a well-known subtype, and Bipolar I Disorder is not caused by an external agent. (*SP 525–527, 530*)

11. **Answer is d.** Sleep disturbances, weight and appetite changes, recurrent thoughts of death and suicide, depressed mood, and loss of pleasure are classic symptoms of depression. These symptoms, or others listed in the diagnostic criteria, must be present almost every day for two weeks to qualify for a diagnosis of Major Depressive Episode. (*SP 524*)

12. **Answer is b.** A gut feeling of dangerousness should never be ignored. Adequate personnel to deal with the patient must be on hand, and once sedated, violent patients must be carefully monitored. If a violent patient specifically threatens certain other people, the physician must inform the potential victims. One should never bargain with violent patients. (*SP 270*)

13. **Answer is c.** Schizophrenic patients show enlargement of the third and lateral ventricles on CT scanning. Cerebrospinal fluid levels of homovanillic acid are high since increased dopamine, and hence its metabolite, is seen to play a role in the genesis of Schizophrenia. The tuberoin-

fundibular tract does not play a role in the pathogenesis of Schizophrenia, but mesolimbic and mesocorticol tracts probably do. Serotonin and norepinephrine play a yet unclear role, and the $D_2$ dopamine receptor seems to play a key role. (*SP 464*)

14. Answer is **c.** The foods ingested by the patient are rich in tyramine, and thus her symptoms are most consistent with her taking a monoamine oxidase inhibitor that has blocked her intestinal metabolism of tyramine and allowed it to enter her bloodstream and act as a pressor. The other medications listed would not have such a reaction. (*SP 974–975*)

15. Answer is **e.** Patients with Neuroleptic Malignant Syndrome are hyperthermic and hypertensive, have muscle rigidity, and are confused. Paranoia is not a part of this clinical picture. (*SP 953*)

16. Answer is **c.** For an acute Manic Episode, the lithium level should be in the range of 0.8 to 1.2 mEq/L. Levels lower than this will be ineffective and higher than this will result in toxicity. (*SP 963*)

17. Answer is **c.** Atrial fibrillation is not associated with the administration of tricyclic antidepressants. A number of electrocardiogram (ECG) changes, including widening of the QRS interval, depression of the ST segment, flattening of the T wave, and tachycardia, are seen in patients taking these medications. (*SP 994*)

18. Answer is **d.** About 10% of patients with Schizophrenia will die as a result of suicide. (*SP 462*)

19. Answer is **b.** Of the list given, being male is the highest risk factor. Persons with Personality Disorders also are somewhat predisposed to suicide. Youth, impulsive attempts, and acting when help is available are lower risk factors. (*SP 809*)

20. Answer is **d.** A positive family history of Schizophrenia, especially in a parent, is a poor prognostic indicator for Schizophrenia. Other symptoms, such as acute onset, affective symptoms, and marriage, are indicators of a better outcome. A clouded sensorium is not associated with the schizophrenic process. (*SP 472*)

21. Answer is **e.** Amantadine is not effective in the treatment of akathisia. Propranolol, benzodiazepine, and clonidine may be more useful. Frequently, this restlessness is confused with an increased psychotic agitation and the dose of antipsychotic is increased, only to worsen the akathisia. Inner anxiety does not play a role in the genesis of this problem. (*SP 950–951*)

22. Answer is **a.** Convulsions would be a later manifestation of lithium toxicity. Ataxia, lethargy, nystagmus, and vom-

iting would all be more common early signs. (*SP 965*)

23. Answer is **d.** The development of cardiac arrhythmias is an ominous sign in the patient with a tricyclic overdose. While the other symptoms listed are serious, this is most likely cause of death with an overdose. (*SP 995*)

24. Answer is **e.** Elderly white people commit suicide at twice the rate of nonwhite people. Chronic illness, alcohol abuse (underestimated in many elderly patients), divorce, and being male are all high risk factors. (*SP 803–804*)

25. Answer is **b.** Bipolar Type II Disorder is characterized by a Hypomanic Episode alternating with Major Depressive Episodes. (*SP 566–568*)

26. Answer is **b.** Hypnagogic hallucinations are hallucinations that occur in the period right before the onset of sleep and are generally thought to be nonpathological. Formication is the hallucinatory process of feeling insects crawling on the skin. Withdrawal from alcohol may produce vivid visual and auditory hallucinations. An illusion is a misinterpretation of a real environmental stimulus. (*SP 307*)

27. Answer is **b.** The death of a spouse is considered to be the greatest stressor humans can experience. Divorce and separation from a spouse are second and third, with jail terms being fourth and death of a close family member fifth. (*SP 755*)

28. Answer is **c.** Of all the symptoms listed, tachycardia is most associated with stress, but although muscle tension, headaches, Anorexia Nervosa, and insomnia are associated with stress as well. (*SP 754*)

29. Answer is **e.** Although the literature on compliance is complex and somewhat confusing, such factors as expense, long waiting times, and lack of continuity of care may affect compliance quite adversely. However, when these factors are controlled, it is still difficult to predict whether a particular patient will be compliant. Patient education and a warm relationship with the physician enhance compliance. (*SP 11–12, 868*)

30. Answer is **d.** Somatic complaints are more common in the depressed elderly patient. Appetite loss with weight loss, fatigue, and sleeplessness would all be usual symptoms in the depressed elderly patient. (*SP 1161*)

31. Answer is **d.** Of the list given the correct order is haloperidol, thiothixene, chlorpromazine. (*SP 956*)

32. Answer is **b.** Good patient education and prompt attention to adverse side effects are very reassuring to patients and enhance compliance. Once-a-day dosing is the most convenient schedule and the most easily remembered by

patients. Even motivated patients will tend to forget to take doses if the frequency of dosing exceeds twice daily. (*SP 11, 865*)

33. Answers are: (1) **a**; (2) **a**; (3) **a**; (4) **c**; (5) **c**; (6) **c**; (7) **c**; (8) **a**; (9) **b**; (10) **b**; (11) **b**; (12) **a**; (13) **b**; (14) **c**; (15) **b**; (16) **b**; (17) **b**; (18) **c**; (19) **c**; (20) **a**. (*SP 948*)

34. Answer is **D**.

35. Answer is **C**.

36. Answer is **B**.

37. Answer is **A**.

38. Answer is **D**.

39. Answer is **A**.

40. Answer is **C**.

41. Answer is **A**.

42. Answer is **A**.

43. Answer is **D**.

44. Answer is **B**.

45. Answer is **A**.

46. Answer is **C**.

47. Answer is **B**.

48. Answer is **B**.

49. Answer is **A**.

50. Answer is **C**.

51. Answer is **A**.

52. Answer is **B**.

53. Answer is **D**.            (*SP 976–981, 991–998*)

54. Answer is **B**.

55. Answer is **C**.

56. Answer is **B**.

57. Answer is **A**.

58. Answer is **B**.

59. Answer is **C**.

60. Answer is **A**.

61. Answer is **B**.

62. Answer is **A**.

63. Answer is **C**.            (*SP 343*)

64. Answer is **a**.

65. Answer is **a**.

66. Answer is **b**.

67. Answer is **b**.

68. Answer is **a**.

69. Answer is **c**.

70. Answer is **c**.

71. Answer is **c**.

72. Answer is **c**.

73. Answer is **a**.            (*SP 586–587, 613*)

74. Answer is **b**.

75. Answer is **a**.

76. Answer is **c**.

77. Answer is **c**.

78. Answer is **b**.

79. Answer is **a**.

80. Answer is **b**.

81. Answer is **a**.

82. Answer is **a**.

83. Answer is **a**.            (*SP 947–953, 976–981, 993–995*)

84. Answer is **g**.

85. Answer is **f**.

86. Answer is **j**.

87. Answer is **h**.

**88.** Answer is **c.**

**89.** Answer is **g.**

**90.** Answer is **a.**

**91.** Answer is **d.**

**92.** Answer is **i.**

**93.** Answer is **k.**

**94.** Answer is **e.**

**95.** Answer is **f.**

**96.** Answer is **a.**

**97.** Answer is **g.**

**98.** Answer is **i.**

**99.** Answer is **c.**

**100.** Answer is **b.**

**101.** Answer is **h.**

**102.** Answer is **f.**

**103.** Answer is **h.**

**104.** Answer is **e.**

**105.** Answer is **d.**

**106.** Answer is **j.**

**107.** Answer is **i.**

**108.** Answer is **b.**

**109.** Answer is **a.**

**110.** Answer is **b.**

**111.** Answer is **b.**

**112.** Answer is **a.**

**113.** Answer is **c.**          *(SP 470–472, 481, 934, 941)*

**114.** Answer is **b.** Alprazolam, imipramine, phenelzine, and fluoxetine have all proved useful in the treatment of Panic Disorder. Thioridazine is not used in the treatment of this disorder. *(SP 589–590)*

**115.** Answer is **c.** Lithium is a simple inorganic salt, abundant in the earth's crust and easily produced and purified for pharmacotherapy. It ionizes in solution and requires 10–12 days to reach complex steady-state equilibrium in total body water. Lithium does not freely cross the blood-brain barrier and CSF levels are 50% of peripheral blood levels. Lithium is almost 100% renally excreted. Hydrochlorothiazide causes lithium retention. Furosemide, a loop diuretic, may cause levels to rise secondary to a concentrating effect, but has little effect on actual excretion. *(SP 966–967)*

**116.** Answer is **e.** Some 20% to 40% of patients with Panic Disorder will have a comorbid Substance Abuse Disorder. Many patients are embarrassed by their symptoms and try to keep them a secret. Half of the patients with this disorder will experience a spontaneous remission if followed long term. Reducing caffeine can significantly reduce symptoms. *(SP 589)*

**117.** Answer is **b.** Located in the rostal pons, the locus ceruleus plays a central role in the mediation of fear and anxiety. It contains most of the noradrenergic cell bodies in the brain, and these neurons project to the limbic system, brain stem, and spinal cord. In nonhuman primates, its ablation results in the inability to form a fear response. It probably receives pain information as a part of its fear-response activity. *(SP 576)*

**118.** Answer is **c.**

**119.** Answer is **a.**

**120.** Answer is **b.**

**121.** Answer is **b.**

**122.** Answer is **a.**

**123.** Answer is **c.**

**124.** Answer is **c.**

**125.** Answer is **a.**

**126.** Answer is **c.**

**127.** Answer is **b.**          *(SP 470–473)*

**128.** Answer is **c.**

**129.** Answer is **a.**

**130.** Answer is **d.**

**131.** Answer is **c.**

**132.** Answer is **b.**

**133.** Answer is **e.**          *(SP 468)*